OPHTHALMOLOGY AND OTOLARYNGOLOGY

for the

Boards and Wards

Other books in the Boards and Wards series:
Boards and Wards — USMLE Steps 2 and 3
Dermatology for the Boards and Wards — USMLE Review
Immunology for the Boards and Wards — USMLE Step 1
Microbiology for the Boards and Wards — USMLE Step 1
Behavioral Sciences and Outpatient Medicine — USMLE Steps 1, 2, and 3
Pathophysiology for the Boards and Wards — USMLE Step 1

OPHTHALMOLOGY AND OTOLARYNGOLOGY

for the

Boards and Wards

Carlos Ayala, MD
Clinical Fellow in Otology and Laryngology
Harvard Medical School
Resident in Otolaryngology
Harvard Otolaryngology Residency Program
Boston, Massachusetts

Brad Spellberg, MD
Resident in Internal Medicine
Harbor-UCLA Medical Center
Torrance, California

b

**Blackwell
Science**

©2002 by Carlos Ayala, Brad Spellberg, and Blackwell Science, Inc.

Editorial Offices:
Commerce Place, 350 Main Street, Malden, Massachusetts 02148, USA
Osney Mead, Oxford OX2 0EL, England
25 John Street, London WC1N 2BL, England
23 Ainslie Place, Edinburgh EH3 6AJ, Scotland
54 University Street, Carlton, Victoria 3053, Australia

Other Editorial Offices:
Blackwell Wissenschafts-Verlag GmbH, Kurfürstendamm 57, 10707 Berlin, Germany
Blackwell Science KK, MG Kodenmacho Building, 7-10 Kodenmacho Nihonbashi, Chuo-ku, Tokyo 104, Japan
Iowa State University Press, A Blackwell Science Company, 2121 S. State Avenue, Ames, Iowa 50014-8300, USA

Distributors:

The Americas
  Blackwell Publishing
  c/o AIDC
  P.O. Box 20
  50 Winter Sport Lane
  Williston, VT 05495-0020
  (Telephone orders: 800-216-2522;
    fax orders: 802-864-7626)
Canada
  Login Brothers Book Company
  324 Saulteaux Crescent
  Winnipeg, Manitoba R3J 3T2
  (Telephone orders: 204-837-2987)

Australia
  Blackwell Science Pty, Ltd.
  54 University Street
  Carlton, Victoria 3053
  (Telephone orders: 03-9347-0300;
    fax orders: 03-9349-3016)
Outside The Americas and Australia
  Blackwell Science, Ltd.
  c/o Marston Book Services, Ltd.
  P.O. Box 269
  Abingdon
  Oxon OX14 4YN
  England
  (Telephone orders: 44-01235-465500;
    fax orders: 44-01235-465555)

Acquisitions: Beverly Copland
Development: Julia Casson
Production: Irene Herlihy
Manufacturing: Lisa Flanagan

Marketing Manager: Toni Fournier
Typeset by Software Services
Printed and bound by Capital City Press

Printed in the United States of America
01 02 03 04 5 4 3 2 1

The Blackwell Science logo is a trade mark of Blackwell Science Ltd., registered at the United Kingdom Trade Marks Registry

Library of Congress Cataloging-in-Publication Data
Ayala, Carlos, MD
    Ophthalmology and otolaryngology for the boards and wards : USMLE steps 1, 2 & 3, / Carlos Ayala, Brad Spellberg.
        p. ; cm.—(Boards and wards series)
    ISBN 0-632-04582-5 (pbk.)
    1. Ophthalmology—Outlines, syllabi, etc. 2. Otolaryngology—Outlines, syllabi, etc.
    [DNLM: 1. Eye Diseases—Outlines. 2. Otorhinolaryngologic Diseases—Outlines. WW 18.2 A9730 2002] I. Title: USMLE steps 1, 2 & 3, ophthalmology and ENT for the boards and wards. II. Spellberg, Brad. III. Title. IV. Series.
    RE50 .A96 2002
    617.7'002'02—dc21

                                                                            2001002391

TABLE OF CONTENTS

PART TWO OTORHINOLARYNGOLOGY (ENT—EAR, NOSE, AND THROAT)

TABLES

FIGURES

COLOR PLATES

ABBREVIATIONS

↑ (↑↑)	increases/high (markedly increases/very high)
↓ (↓↓)	decreases/low (markedly decreases/very low)
→	causes/leads to/analysis shows
1°/2°	primary/secondary
BP	blood pressure
Bx	biopsy
CA	carcinoma
CN	cranial nerve
CNS	central nervous system
CXR/X-ray	chest x-ray/x-ray
Dx/DDx	differential diagnosis
ETOH	ethyl alcohol
dz	disease
HA	headache
HTN	hypertension
Hx/FHx	history/family history
ICP	intracranial pressure
I&D	incision and drainage
infxn	infection
IVIG	intravenous immunoglobulin
N or Nml	normal
PE	physical exam or pulmonary embolus
pt(s)	patient(s)
Px	prognosis
Si/Sx/aSx	sign/symptom/asymptomatic
subQ	subcutaneous
Tx	treatment/therapy
Utz	ultrasound

PREFACE

Based on the positive feedback about the Head and Neck and Ophthalmology section in our first Boards & Wards books, we decided to develop a freestanding concise medical student reference book.

We reviewed the lists of testable topics on the USMLE steps 1, 2, and 3 and added to this information various clinical correlates and observations to enhance the presentation of this high yield book. We maintain our outline format in order to spare readers needless information and to save time for busy medical students and interns who need a quick, ready reference for review.

ACKNOWLEDGMENTS & CONTRIBUTORS

Special thanks to all those involved in the development of this book, most especially the following people who directly contributed their time and wisdom in the review of the manuscript.

Lynnette M. Watkins, MD
Director Emergency Ophthalmology Service
Staff Physician, Ophthalmic Plastic Surgery
Instructor in Ophthalmology, Harvard Medical School

Ramon Arturo Franco, Jr., MD
Department of Otology and Laryngology
Harvard Medical School
Fellow, Division of Laryngology, MEEI

Mitchell Ramsey, MD
Department of Otology and Laryngology
Harvard Medical School
Fellow, Division of Otology, MEEI

Kenneth Whittemore, MD
Chief Resident
Harvard Otolaryngology Residency Program
Department of Otology and Laryngology
Harvard Medical School

FIGURE CREDITS

Figures 1, 2, 4, 5, 6, 7, 8, 9, 10, 11, 12, 13, 14, 15, 16, 17 reproduced with permission from James B, Chew C, Bron A. *Lecture Notes on Ophthalmology*, 8th ed. Oxford, UK: Blackwell Science, 1997.

Figures 18, 19, 20, 22, 23, 24, 25, 28, 29, 30, 31, 32, 33, 34 reproduced with permission from Bull PD. *Lecture Notes on Diseases of the Ear, Nose and Throat*, 8th ed. Oxford, UK: Blackwell Science, 1996.

Figure 3 reproduced with permission from Pritchard TC, Alloway KD. *Medical Neuroscience*. Madison, CT: Fence Creek Publishing, 1999.

Figures 26, 27 reproduced with permission from Axford J. *Medicine*. Blackwell Science, 1996.

Figure 21 reproduced with permission from Armstrong P, Wastie ML. *Diagnostic Imaging*, 4th ed. Oxford, UK: Blackwell Science, 1998.

PART ONE

OPHTHALMOLOGY

I. BASIC EMBRYOLOGY

A. Eye Embryology (Table 1)

TABLE 1 Eye Embryology	
ADULT STRUCTURE	**DEVELOPMENTAL DERIVATION**
Retina, retinal pigment epithelium, ciliary epithelium, iris epithelium	Optic cup-(neuroectoderm) ectoderm derived from neural tube
Optic nerve	Optic stalk + optic axons-(neuroectoderm)
Lens, anterior corneal epithelium, lacrimal glands, lacrimal drainage apparatus, conjunctival epithelium, caruncle, lids, cilia	Surface ectoderm
Sclera (superotemporally) extraocular muscles (fibres), endothelium of blood vessels, vitreous	Mesoderm
Central retinal artery & vein	Hyaloid artery & vein (mesoderm)
Iris*	Iris sphincter and dilator-neuroectoderm, iris stroma-neural crest cells
Corneal stroma and endothelium, sclera, choroid, ciliary muscle, orbital bones, orbital fat, connective tissue trabecular meshwork, orbital bones, connective tissue of orbit	Neural crest cells

* Clinical Note: Coloboma iridis—Cleft or notch in iris commonly associated with a failure of choroid fissure closure.
May extend to ciliary body, retina, or optic nerve.
May be associated with CHARGE or other eye defects (see CHARGE Associations).

B. Ocular Embryological Time Table (Table 2)

TABLE 2	Ocular Embryological Timetable
Day 23	Optic pit forms
Day 25	Optic vesicle forms
Day 27	Optic vesicle induces lens placode
Day 33	Embryonic fissure closes (failure of fissure closure—coloboma formation)
Second month	• Eyelid folds appear • Retinal differentiation begins • Neural crest cells of corneal endothelium migrate, then corneal stroma • Axons from ganglion cells migrate to optic nerve
Third month	• Rod and cone precursors form • Eyelids meet and fuse • Ciliary body develops
Fourth month	• Hyaloid system regresses • Retinal vessels grow • Iris sphincter develops
Fifth month	• Eyelids separate • Photoreceptors differentiate
Sixth month	• Iris dilator develops • Ganglion cells thicken in macula
Seventh month	• Choroid obtains pigmentation • Fovea forms
Eighth month	• Anterior chamber completes formation • Hyaloid system disappears
Ninth month	• Retinal vessels reach periphery • Optic nerve myelination complete to lamina cribosa

II. ANATOMY (see Figure 1)

A. Eyeball (Globe)

1. Volume of globe 6.5 cc

2. Three layers of the eye

   a. Corneal/scleral layer

ANATOMY OF THE EYE

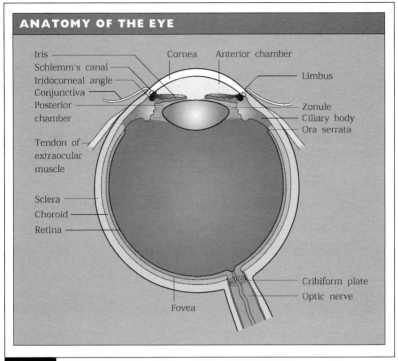

The Basic Anatomy of the Eye

    b. Uvea (iris, ciliary body, choroid)

    c. Retina (neurosensory retina, retinal pigment epithelium)

B. Conjunctiva

1. Mucous membrane

2. Contains goblet cells important in mucus formation and tear film production

3. Lines the globe (bulbar), posterior lids (palpebral), and fornix (forniceal)

C. Cornea

1. Air/tear film/cornea interface main refractive area of the eye

2. Consists of epithelium, Bowman's layer and stroma, Descemet's membrane, and endothelium

3. Collagen and glycosaminoglycans main components of the cornea

D. Iris

1. Consists of iris stroma, blood vessels, iris sphincter, and dilator muscle

2. Attaches to ciliary body at iris root

3. Iris sphincter innervated by parasympathetics

4. Iris dilator innervated by sympathetics

E. Lens

1. Second refractive area of the eye

2. Consists of lens fibers, lens epithelium, and lens sutures

3. Lens zonules hold the lens in place

4. Lacks innervation and vascularization

5. Aqueous and vitreous provide nourishment

F. Ciliary Body

1. Consists of epithelium and stroma

2. Forms the aqueous humor

3. Ciliary muscle important in accommodation (changing the shape of the lens to aid in near vision)

4. Tear between the longitudinal and circular muscle seen in angle recession

G. Aqueous Humor

1. Optically clear fluid without cells, protein

2. High in ascorbate

3. Formed by ciliary body

H. Sclera

1. Tough outer coating of the eye

2. Consists of collagen, elastin

3. Thinnest areas of sclera at limbus, muscle insertions

4. The most common site of rupture or open globe injury

I. Choroid

1. Fibrovascular layer with pigmentation
2. Supports the outer layer of the retina
3. Highest blood flow rate in the body
4. Important component in the blood–ocular barrier

J. Retina (see Figure 2)

1. Consists of photoreceptors (rods and cones), support cells and axons, ganglion cells, nerve fiber layer, and blood vessels
2. Macula is the area responsible for central vision, has largest concentration of cones and more than one layer of ganglion cells

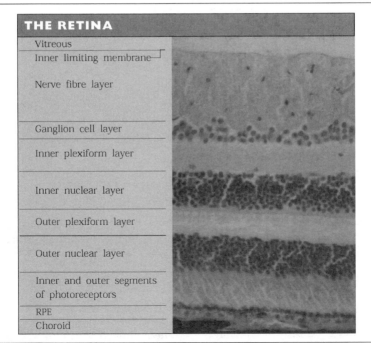

THE RETINA

Vitreous
Inner limiting membrane
Nerve fibre layer
Ganglion cell layer
Inner plexiform layer
Inner nuclear layer
Outer plexiform layer
Outer nuclear layer
Inner and outer segments of photoreceptors
RPE
Choroid

FIGURE 2 The Structure of the Retina

3. Blood supply of inner retina from central retinal artery, outer retina supplied by the choriocapillaris portion of the choroid

4. Retinal pigment epithelium supports the neurosensory retina

K. Vitreous Humor

1. Consists of collagen and hyaluronic acid

2. Attaches to the lens, optic disc, fovea, and base

3. Shrinks and loses water content as aging process continues

L. Optic Nerve

1. Consists of axons from retinal ganglion cells

2. Longest portion of the optic nerve is intraorbital

3. Blood supply from ophthalmic artery, pial arteries, central retinal artery, and ciliary arteries

M. Orbital Vault

1. Orbital volume 30 cc

2. Osteology

   a. Roof of orbit—frontal and lesser wing of sphenoid

   b. Lateral wall—greater wing of sphenoid, zygoma

   c. Floor—maxilla, palatine, zygomatic

   d. Medial wall—ethmoid, lacrimal, maxilla, sphenoid

   e. Weakest part of the orbit is posteriomedial orbital floor

   f. Strongest part of the orbit is lateral wall

   g. Contains globe, orbital fat, vessels, nerves, and extraocular muscles

   h. Continuous with the superior and inferior orbital fissures, optic foramen

N. Eyelids

1. Form of barrier protection for the globe

2. Consists of skin, muscle, fat, fascia, and tarsus (fibrous connective tissue)

3. Tarsus is main support structure of eyelid

4. Orbicularis main protractor of eyelids

5. Levator superioris main retractor of upper eyelid, lower lid retractors less well defined

O. Extraocular Muscles

1. Rectus muscles (superior, lateral, inferior, medial)

   a. Medial—adduction

   b. Lateral—abduction

   c. Superior—elevation, adduction, and intortion

   d. Inferior—depression, adduction, and extortion

2. Oblique muscles (superior, inferior)

   a. Superior— intortion, abduction, and depression

   b. Inferior—extortion, abduction, and elevation

3. All innervated by cranial nerve III except lateral rectus (cranial nerve VI) and superior oblique (cranial nerve IV)

4. Spiral of Tillaux—imaginary line connecting insertions of recti muscle

5. All rectus muscles except the lateral rectus have dual blood vessel supply

P. Lacrimal Drainage System

1. Includes the puncta, canaliculi, lacrimal sac, and nasolacrimal duct

2. Most common area of obstruction is the nasolacrimal duct

3. Nasolacrimal duct drains below the inferior turbinate in the nose

Q. Lacrimal Gland

1. Sits in the lacrimal fossa of the frontal bone

2. Has two lobes—orbital and palpebral

3. Removal of the palpebral lobe causes dry eye

4. Responsible for reflex tearing

III. LOSS OF VISION

A. Neuropathology

1. **Unexplained Visual Loss**—optic nerve disorders

   a. **Prechiasmal (see Figure 3)**

      1) Can see disc edema with elevation and blurred disc margins

      2) May have central, altitudinal, and arcuate scotomas

      3) Afferent pupillary defect (Marcus-Gunn pupil)

         a) Due to afferent defect of CN II, pupil will not react to direct light but will react consensually when light is directed at the normal contralateral eye

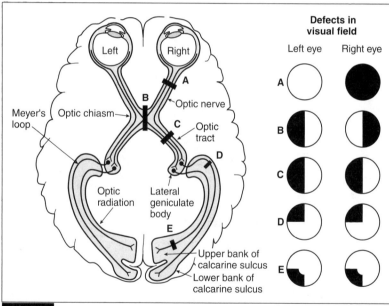

FIGURE 3 **Visual Field Deficits**

Lesions in the visual system are correlated with specific visual field deficits. (A) Blindness in the right eye. (B) Bitemporal heteronymous hemianopsia. (C) Left homonymous hemianopsia. (D) Superior quadrantic anopia. (E) Inferior quadrantic anopsia with macular sparing. (Reproduced with permission from Pritchard TC and Alloway KD. Medical Neuroscience. *Madison, CT: Fence Creek Publishing, 1999:307. ©Fence Creek Publishing, LLC.)*

b) **Characterized by swinging flashlight test**

   i) Swing penlight quickly back & forth between eyes

   ii) Denervated pupil will not constrict to direct stimulation & **instead will actually appear to dilate when light is shone in it** because it is dilating back to baseline when consensual light is removed from other eye

4) Categories

  a) Optic neuritis

    i) Idiopathic inflammation of optic nerve

    ii) Often seen in demyelinating disease—multiple sclerosis

    iii) Acute monocular vision loss of variable severity

    iv) Pain upon eye movement

    v) Vision improves within 2–8 wk

    vi) **Funduscopic exam reveals disk hyperemia or may be normal**

    vii) Tx observation vs. intravenous corticosteroids

  b) Retrobulbar neuritis "the patient sees nothing—the physician sees nothing"

  c) Ischemic optic neuropathy

    i) Acute severe vision loss with minimal resolution over time

    ii) Nonarteritic anterior ischemic optic neuropathy

      a)) Unilateral disc edema

      b)) Central or altitudinal visual field defect

      c)) Seen in patients with hypertension or diabetes

      d)) Vascular etiology

      e)) Poor final visual acuity

      f)) Affects other eye in 30% of patients

    iii) Arteritic ischemic optic neuropathy (temporal arteritis)

      a)) Granulomatous inflammation of medium size arteries

        b)) Incidence increases with age

        c)) Also have weight loss, fatigue, scalp tenderness, jaw claudication, and muscle and joint pain

        d)) High sedimentation rate

    d) Compressive optic neuropathy—slowly progressive painless loss of vision

      i) Optic nerve glioma—seen in children and neurofibromatosis

      ii) Optic nerve sheath meningioma

        a)) Seen in middle-aged women

        b)) Vision loss, optic atrophy, and shunt vessels on optic disc are classic triad

    e) Infiltrative optic neuropathy

      i) Inflammatory—sarcoidosis

      ii) Infectious—syphilis, tuberculosis, toxoplasmosis

      iii) Neoplastic—leukemia, lymphoma, carcinomatosis

      iv) Leukemic involvement requires urgent radiation therapy to save vision

    f) Radiation optic neuropathy may occur years after radiation exposure

    g) Traumatic optic neuropathy

    h) Toxic/metabolic optic neuropathy

    i) Hereditary optic neuropathy

  b. **Chiasmal disorders**

    1) Have visual fields deficits

    2) Bitemporal hemianopsia (unable to see bilateral temporal fields)

      a) Causes

        i) Pituitary adenoma

        ii) Craniopharyngioma

        iii) Meningioma

        iv) Aneurysm

        v) Trauma

c. **Postchiasmal disorders**

   1) Occiptal cortex lesions

      a) From stroke, tumor, and vascular malformations

      b) Congrous homonymous hemianopia (unable to see on same side in both eyes)

   2) Temporal lobe lesions

      a) From tumor

      b) "Pie in the sky" visual field deficits

      c) Also see seizures, formed visual hallucinations

   3) Parietal lobe lesions

      a) Also from tumor, stroke

      b) Also can see neglect, agraphia, agnosia

      c) Inferior quandrantinopia "pie on the floor" visual field deficit

IV. CLASSIC SYNDROMES AND SYMPTOMS

A. Eye Disorders

1. Diplopia (double vision)

   a. Monocular (present when one eye is closed), commonly caused by cataracts

   b. Binocular (both eyes open)—occurs when both eyes are not fixed on the same point

      1) Cranial nerve palsies

         a) CN III

            i) Loss of adduction, elevation, and/or depression

            ii) Seen in trauma, tumor (aneurysm), post-viral infection, and microvascular disease (hypertension)

            iii) Partial or pupil-involving third nerve palsies— must evaluate for aneurysm

         b) CN IV

            i) Most often seen after trauma, but also congenital or microvascular disease

        ii) Binocular vertical diplopia

        iii) Patients have head tilt to side opposite lesion

    c) CN VI

        i) Loss of abduction

        ii) Binocular horizontal diplopia worse at distance

        iii) Post-viral, tumor, trauma, microvascular disease in children

        iv) Multiple sclerosis, tumor, increased intracranial pressure in adults

        v) If palsy bilateral or present more than three months—neuroimaging indicated to evaluate for tumor

  c. Other causes of diplopia

    1) Thyroid ophthalmopathy (Graves ophthalmopathy) seen commonly on upward gaze because of inflammatory infiltration of inferior rectus

    2) Myasthenia gravis

      a) Progressively worsening diplopia, may be preceded by ptosis

      b) Symptoms improve with edrophonium (Tensilon diagnostic test)

  d. Orbital fracture causes upward gaze impairment by entrapment of extraocular muscles, usually inferior rectus or medial rectus

2. Eye movement disorders

  a. Horizontal

    1) Ocular motor apraxia

      a) Inability to initiate saccades

      b) Bilateral frontoparietal lesions

      c) Patients "whip" their heads abruptly to turn eye

    2) Internuclear ophthalmoplegia

      a) Classically found in multiple sclerosis, also in stroke and pontine tumor, aneurysm

      b) Lesion is located in the median longitudinal fasciculus (MLF)

      c) Causes inability to adduct the ipsilateral eye past midline on lateral gaze with abduction nystagmus of the contralateral eye (inability to perform conjugate gaze), diplopia

      d) Caused by lack of communication between contralateral CN VI nucleus & the ipsilateral CN III nucleus

      e) Can be unilateral or bilateral

      f) Symptoms include binocular horizontal diplopia, ocular flutter, opsoclonus = wild multidirectional eye movements, seen in neuroblastoma

  b. Vertical

    1) Parinaud's (dorsal midbrain) syndrome

      a) Midbrain tectum lesion with bilateral paralysis of upward gaze

      b) Commonly associated with pineal tumor, stroke, arteriovenous malformation, and demyelinating disease

      c) Also see light-near dissociation of pupil function, lid retraction, and convergence-retraction nystagmus

    2) Progressive supranuclear palsy

      a) Degenerative neurologic disorder with progressive deterioration of voluntary eye movements

      b) Downgaze affected first

      c) Also see axial rigidity, dementia, and dysarthria

B. Eyelid Disturbances

1. Ptosis

  a. Seen with third nerve palsy, Horner's syndrome, and myasthenia gravis

  b. Myasthenia gravis

    1) Neuromuscular disorder causing muscle weakness

    2) Seen predominantly in females

    3) Variable ptosis (worse in evening), diplopia

    4) Associated with thyroid disease, autoimmune diseases

2. Lid retraction seen with Graves ophthalmopathy, dorsal midbrain (Parinaud's) syndrome

3. Anisocoria (unequal pupil size)

   a. Physiologic

      1) Seen in 20% of normal patients

      2) Usually less than 1 mm difference

   b. Abnormally dilated pupils

      1) Third nerve palsy

         a) Pupillomotor fibers from Edinger–Westfall nucleus on peripheral portion of third nerve, vulnerable to compression from tumor, ANEURYSM, and trauma

         b) Traumatic mydriasis caused by tears of the iris sphincter after trauma, leading to unimpeded dilation

         c) Pharmacologic mydriasis caused by drops that dilate the pupil and/or paralyze the ciliary muscle (e.g., atropine)

         d) Adie's tonic pupil

            i) Dilated pupil with light near dissociation, slow constriction, and redilation

            ii) Caused by abnormal function of the ciliary ganglion and denervation hypersensitivity

            iii) Usually in females

            iv) 70% of patients have absent deep tendon reflex (Adie syndrome)

            v) Pharmocologic testing with different strengths of pilocarpine to establish diagnosis

               a)) Adie pupil will constrict to dilute pilocarpine (1/8%)

               b)) Pharmacologic mydriasis will not respond to full strength pilocarpine

   c. Abnormally small (miotic) pupils

      1) Horner's syndrome

a) Caused by sympathetic innervation damage anywhere along pathway from hypothalamus to spinal cord to superior cervical ganglion to iris dilator muscle

b) Etiologies include stroke, mediastinal mass, Pancoast's tumor, neck trauma or surgery, carotid dissection, or congenital

c) Also associated with ptosis, anhidrosis (absence of sweating)

d) Congenital form associated with iris heterochromia (eye color lighter on involved side)

e) **Note: Pharmacologic pupil testing with cocaine and hydroxyamphetamine to establish and locate lesion**

   i) Cocaine blocks reuptake of norepinephrine—if pupil does not dilate, it is a Horner's

   ii) Hydroxyamphetamine stimulates release of norepinephrine from nerve terminals—if the pupil dilates, the Horner is a preganglionic Horner's pupil (more serious), if it does not dilate, the pupil is a postganglionic Horner's pupil

2) Argyll-Robertson pupil

   a) Small irregular pupil

   b) Bilateral, pupils accommodate but don't react to light

   c) Associated with tertiary syphilis

3) Pharmacologic miosis caused by cholinomimetics or opioids

4) Iritis causes small pupil secondary to inflammation and synechiae (scarring) between the iris and lens

4. **Nystagmus**

   a. Involuntary, rhythmic oscillation of eyes with a fast and slow component. Fast component of nystagmus identifies type

   b. May be caused by peripheral or central vestibular lesion

  d. Peripheral nystagmus can be inhibited by fixation of eyes. It is usually unidirectional, horizontal, or torsional in nature. It can be caused by lesions affecting the labyrinth or semicircular canals

  e. Central nystagmus is not inhibited by fixation of eyes, may change direction, commonly vertical in nature. Caused by lesions affecting the brain stem and cerebellum

  f. Downbeat nystagmus associated with cervicomedullary junction lesions

  g. Assess patient with attention to drug history

  h. May need MRI if unexplainable recent onset

V. PEDIATRIC OPHTHALMOLOGY AND STRABISMUS

A. Amblyopia

1. Decreased vision secondary to failure of development of the pathway between the retina and visual cortex before age 7 in an anatomically normal eye

2. Types of amblyopia

  a. Refractive (one eye more near- or far-sighted than the other, or both very near- or very far-sighted)

  b. Occlusion (secondary to cataract, ptosis, tumor)

  c. Strabismic (abnormal turning of one eye or other)

   1) Unilateral or bilateral

   2) Tx = correct refractive error, patching, cataract or lid surgery to correct occlusion, strabismus surgery to realign eyes

B. Strabismus (Ocular Misalignment)

1. Normal alignment is termed orthotropia

2. Congenital or acquired

3. Esotropia—an inturning ocular misalignment (inwardly rotated "crossed eyes")

  a. Often associated with refractive error (hyperopia)

  b. Congenital esotropia has largest amount of deviation

    c. Amount of convergence during accomodation may be high

4. Exotropia—an outward deviation of ocular alignment (outwardly rotated "walled eyes")

    a. Often after sensory deprivation

    b. Amblyopia rare

5. Hypertropia—eye deviated up, often seen in fourth nerve palsy, thyroid orbitopathy, myasthenia gravis

6. Hypotropia—eye deviated down

C. Congenital Cataracts

1. Opacity of the lens from birth

2. Cataracts greater than 3 mm in size increase risk of occlusion amblyopia

3. Polar, sutural, nuclear, lamellar, zonular types

4. Causes

    a. Chromosomal abnormalities (Down, Turner, Lowe syndromes)

    b. Infections (rubella, varicella, toxoplasmosis, syphilis)

    c. Metabolic (galactosemia, hypocalcemia)

    d. Birth trauma

    e. Most unilateral cases not metabolic or genetic

5. Treatment is surgical in cases where ambyopia is a risk

D. Congenital Glaucoma

1. Bilateral

    a. Male

    b. Classic triad = tearing, photophobia, blepharospasm

    c. Associated with Sturge-Weber, Lowe oculocerebrorenal syndrome, Marfan syndrome

    d. Si/Sx = decreased vision, corneal edema, increased intraocular pressure, large (bupthalmic) eye

    e. Treatment is surgical

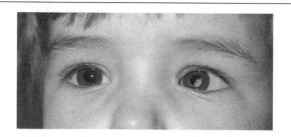

FIGURE 4 Left Leukocoria

E. Leukocoria (see Figure 4)

1. Group of disorders in infants or children that cause pupil to look white

2. Associated with eye turn, decreased vision, and abnormality of globe size

3. Anterior segment—cataract

4. Posterior segment

   a. Retinoblastoma

   b. Coats disease (exudative retinopathy with telangiectasias)

   c. Retinopathy of prematurity

   d. Toxoplasmosis

   e. Toxocariasis

   f. Coloboma (defect of choroid, iris, due to failure of fusion of embryonic fissure)

   g. Persistent hyperplastic primary vitreous

   h. Retinal detachment

VI. CORNEA AND EXTERNAL DISEASES

A. External Disease

1. Pterygium (see Figure 5 and Color Plate 1)

   a. Fleshy fibrovascular tissue growth from conjunctiva onto nasal side of cornea

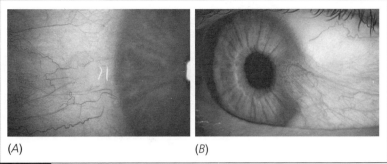

(A)   (B)

FIGURE 5

The clinical appearance of (A) a pingueculum; (B) a pterygium.

   b. Associated with exposure to wind, sand, sun, and dust

   c. Tx = cosmetic removal unless impairing vision lubrication if inflammed

2. Pinguecula

   a. Benign yellowish nodules on either side of the cornea

   b. Tx = observation, lubrication if becomes irritated

B. Cornea

1. Corneal abrasion (see Figure 6 and Color Plate 2)

   a. Often results from direct trauma to eye

   b. Pain, tearing, and photophobia are present

   c. Dx = fluorescein to stain areas of corneal defect

   d. Tx = topical antibiotics & oral analgesics

   e. Cornea usually heals in 24–48 hr, should reexamine pt the next day

   f. Patient at risk for recurrent erosion syndrome—repetitive sloughing of the corneal epithelium due to lack of firm adhesion to Bowman's layer

2. Corneal ulceration

   a. Due to bacteria, fungi, amoebae, or viruses

   b. Often occurs in contact lens wearers (*Pseudomonas*, Acanthoamoeba)

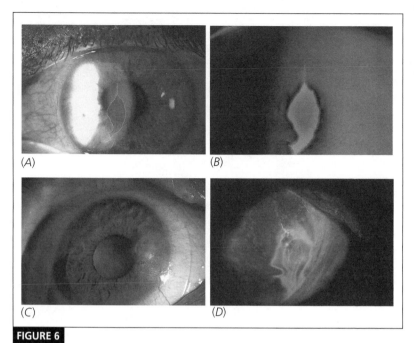

(A) (B)
(C) (D)

FIGURE 6

*(A) A corneal abrasion (the corneal epithelial layer has been damaged).
(B) Fluorescein uniformly stains the area of damage. (C) A perforated cornea leaking aqueous (the leak is protected here with a soft contact lens).
(D) The fluorescein fluoresces as it is diluted by the leaking aqueous.*

  c. Dense infiltrate with epithelial defect staining with fluorescein dye, pain/photophobia may be minimal

  d. **Hypopyon (pus in anterior chamber) is a grave sign**

  e. Healing of ulcer leads to scarring that can impair vision

  f. **This is an emergency! Get ophthalmology consult now!**

 3. Keratitis (inflammation of cornea)

  a. Viral

   1) Acute keratitis usually caused by adenovirus or HSV

   2) **Herpes simplex shows characteristic dendritic branching on fluorescein staining**

   3) Multiple recurrences lead to corneal anesthesia, ulceration, permanent scarring, and possible perforation

   4) Tx = topical antiviral: vidarabine or idoxuridine

b. Bacterial/parasitic

1) Often caused by extended wear contact lenses, poor lens hygiene, corneal trauma

2) Most common pathogens are *Pseudomonas aeruginosa, S. pneumonia, Moraxella spp., & Staph. spp.*

3) Corneal culture and broad spectrum topical antibiotics (e.g., quinolones)

4) **This is an emergency! Get ophthalmology consult now!**

C. Red Eye (see Figures 7 and 8 and Color Plate 3)

1. Assess pain, visual acuity, type of eye discharge, and pupillary abnormalities in all patients

2. Immediate ophthalmology consult if sx persist, worsen, or unsure of diagnosis

3. Common ophthalmic disorders presenting as **Red Eye** (Table 3)

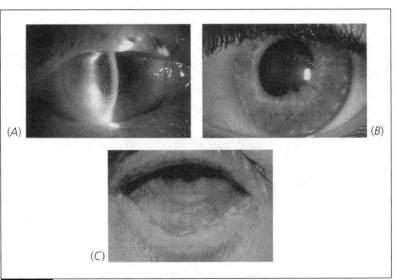

(A)

(B)

(C)

FIGURE 7   **Signs of Anterior Uveitis**

(A) Keratics precipitates on the corneal endothelium. (B) Posterior synechiae (adhesions between the lens and iris) give the pupil an irregular appearance. (C) A hypopyon, white cells have collected as a mass in the inferior anterior chamber.

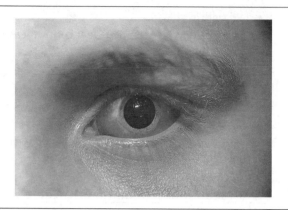

FIGURE 8   A Subconjunctival Hemorrhage

D. Episcleritis/Scleritis

1. Episcleritis

   a. Inflammation of the episcleral vessels (vessels blanch with topcial phenylephrine)

   b. Sectoral or diffuse, may be nodular

   c. Most often idiopathic and self-limited

   d. More often associated with systemic disease if recurrent or bilateral (rheumatoid arthritis, syphilis, TB, herpes zoster)

2. Scleritis

   a. Extremely painful, red, photophobic eyes

   b. Often associated with collagen-vascular disease (rheumatoid arthritis, lupus, Wegener's granulomatosis), infection (syphilis, TB)

   c. Thinned sclera with bluish hue

   d. Risk of perforation of sclera, resulting in loss of the eye

   e. Tx = **systemic** prednisone, nonsteroidals, immunosuppressive agents

E. Uveitis

1. Defined as inflammation of the iris, ciliary body, and/or choroid (all layers form the uvea)

2. Granulomatous (e.g., sarcoidosis) or nongranulomatous (e.g., juvenile rheumatoid arthritis)

TABLE 3	Common Ophthalmic Disorders Presenting as Red Eye		
DISEASE	**Si/Sx**	**CAUSE**	**Tx**
Bacterial conjunctivitis	Significant pain, purulent discharge, no pupillary changes	• *S. pneumoniae, Staph spp., N. gonorrhoeae, Chlamydia trachomatis, H. influenzae*	• Gram stain and cultures, topical polysporin, erythromycin, quinolones
Viral conjunctivitis	Minimal pain and itching, no vision changes (unless keratitis present), watery discharge, no pupillary changes. Preauricular adenopathy. Often associated with pharyngitis (adenovirus)	• Adenovirus most common others— HSV, varicella, EBV, influenza, echovirus, coxsackie virus	• Self-limiting, very contagious • Ophthalmology consult for late sequelae, scarring
Allergic conjunctivitis	Moderate to severe itching, foreign body sensation, dryness. Tearing, chemosis (marked edema of conjunctiva)	• Environmental allergens, medicamentosa	• Antihistamine, mast cell stabilizer, or steroid drops (in severe cases)
Xerophthalmia (dry eye)	Foreign body sensation, blurriness, no pupillary changes, no discharge. Bitot's spots (desquamated, keratinized conjunctival cells) seen in vitamin A deficiency	• Sjogren's disease (Keratoconjuctivitis sicca) • Vitamin A deficiency Dx—Schirmer test—place filter paper over conjunctival surface of eyelid with (or without) anesthetic to measure basal tearing (basal and reflex tearing without anesthetic)	• Artificial tears and ointment • Vitamin A, punctal plugs, or cautery to decrease tear outflow or loss

TABLE 3	*Continued*		
DISEASE	**Si/Sx**	**CAUSE**	**Tx**
Corneal abrasion	Painful, with photophobia, tearing, blurriness	• Direct trauma to eye, fingernail, tree branch, rose bush, contact lens, etc. • Dx by slit lamp exam and fluorescein stain to detect areas of corneal defect	• Antibiotics, examine daily. NO PATCHING if injury secondary to vegetative matter or foreign body
Keratitis	Pain, photophobia, tearing, decreased vision hypopyon-pus in anterior chamber is a grave sign	• Corneal infection adenovirus, HSV, *S. pneumoniae*, *Moraxella*, Staph., *Pseudomonas* (contact lens users) herpes shows classic dendritic branching on fluorescein or rose bengal stain	• Emergency, immediate • Ophtho consult • Topical antibiotics or • Antivirals
Uveitis (Figure 7)	Inflammation of the iris, ciliary body, and/or choroid. Pain, miosis, photophobia. Flare (proteinaceous debris) & white blood cells seen in aqueous humor on slit lamp examination	• Seen in seronegative spondyloarthro-pathy, inflammatory bowel dz, sarcoidosis, infxn (CMV, syphilis), autoimmune disease (lupus, rheumatoid arthritis)	• Treat underlying disease, topical or po steroids, cycloplegics

TABLE 3	*Continued*		
DISEASE	**Si/Sx**	**CAUSE**	**Tx**
Angle closure glaucoma	Severe pain, blurry vision, halos around lights. Fixed mid-dilated pupil. Globe tender to palpation	• ↓ aqueous humor outflow because of obstruction of angle by peripheral iris. Can be exacerbated by mydriatics. Must examine both eyes, other eye usually also has a narrow angle	• Emergency! Topical and oral acetazolamide, topical aqueous suppressants, miotics, laser iridotomy for cure
Subconjunctival hemorrhage (Figure 8)	Spontaneous onset of painless bright red patch on sclera caused by rupture of episcleral vessel	• Overexertion, valsalva, or trauma. Can also be seen in patients with uncontrolled hypertension	• Self-limited • Check blood pressure

3. Sx = hazy vision, black floating spots, pain & photophobia, ciliary injection, miotic pupil, increased or decreased intraocular pressure, keratic precipitates, hypopyon (white blood cells layered in the anterior chamber), cataract, macular edema

4. Retinal detachment & glaucoma can be late sequelae of disease

5. Anterior, intermediate, posterior uveitis—panuveitis involves all of these areas

6. Associated systemic diseases

   a. Autoimmune diseases: ankylosing spondylitis, Reiter's syndrome, Behçet's syndrome, lupus, & sarcoidosis

   b. Infections—toxoplasmosis, CMV, toxocariasis, histoplasmosis, TB, syphilis

   c. Inflammatory bowel disease, psoriatic arthritis

7. Masquerade syndromes mimic uveitis and include—retinoblastoma, large cell lymphoma, intraocular foreign body, and melanoma

8. **Chorioretinitis**

   a. Posterior uveitis affecting the retina

   b. Usually follows an active microbial invasion of the tissues by most commonly toxoplasma gondii

   c. Can occur in utero

   d. Si/Sx = blurred vision, photophobia, pupil is often constricted and/or irregular in shape

   e. Lesions appear as yellowish-white patches through a hazy vitreous

   f. Tx = ophthalmology consult, antibiotics, and systemic corticosteroids

   g. Prognosis: If the macular area was not involved, central acuity remains normal

F. <u>Glaucoma (see Figure 9 and Color Plate 4)</u>

1. Progressive optic neuropathy with characteristic visual field loss often (not always) related to increased intraocular pressure

2. Major cause of blindness in the aging (leading cause of blindness in African Americans)

3. Can be open or closed type

   a. Open-angle glaucoma

      1) Causation unknown, mechanical vs. vascular vs. toxic (glutamate) theory

      2) Rarely causes pain or corneal edema

      3) Constriction of visual field in later stages

      4) Incidence increases with age

      5) On funduscopic examination, classic finding increases in size of optic cup with thinning of neural rim

      6) Tx

         a) Medical = cholinergics, alpha-agonists, beta-blockers, carbonic anhydrase inhibitors prostaglandin analogue

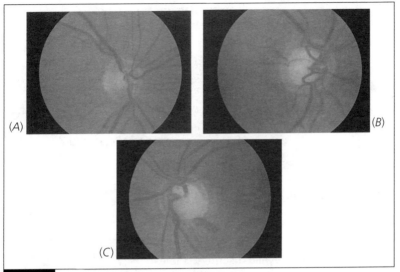

FIGURE 9

Comparison of (A) a normal optic disc; (B) glaucomatous optic disc; (C) a disc hemorrhage is a feature of patients with low-tension glaucoma.

  b) Laser surgery to stretch trabecular meshwork and facilitate outflow

  c) Surgery to facilitate alternate drainage pathway for aqueous

b. Angle-closure glaucoma

  1) Can be chronic or acute, the latter is an emergency

  2) Typically idiopathic, can be drug induced (mydriatics)

  3) Mydriatics cause the peripheral iris to move forward & occlude the aqueous fluid outflow tract

  4) Prodromal Sx = sudden pain in eye & head, halos around lights, blurry vision

  5) Acute attack causes severe throbbing pain in eye, radiating to CN V distribution, blurry vision, nausea/vomiting, fixed, mid-dilated pupil, redness

  6) This is considered an emergency because blindness can occur

  7) Tx

    a) iv or oral acetazolamide, topical timolol, pilocarpine (stretches and pulls the iris away from the angle)

    b) Mydriatics NOT recommended (can exacerbate condition)—laser iridotomy follows to establish alternate pathway for aqueous to flow allowing iris to bow back into position

    c) Laser iridotomy indicated in asymptomatic eye to prevent future occurrence of angle closure

VII. LIDS/LACRIMAL/ORBIT

A. Lids

1. **Common eyelid disorders** (Table 4)

B. Lacrimal

1. **Congenital nasolacrimal duct obstruction**

   a. Secondary to imperforate membrane at the valve of Hasner (exit of the nasolacrimal duct)

   b. Spontaneously resolves in the first nine months with massage and antibiotics

   c. Remainder will need probing and irrigation, other surgical intervention

2. **Nasolacrimal duct obstruction**

   a. Congenital or acquired

       1) Acquired disease secondary to chronic sinus disease, facial trauma, involutional stenosis (older adults), dacryocystitis, granulomatous disease (Wegener's, sarcoidosis)

       2) Tearing, crusting, discharge, recurrent conjunctivitis

       3) Tx = intubation of nasolacrimal duct system, surgery for anastomosis between tear sac and nasal cavity (dacryocystorhinostomy)

3. **Dacryocystitis** (see Figure 10)

   a. Acute or chronic infection of lacrimal sac, usually caused by *Staphylococcus aureus*, *Streptococcus pneumoniae*,

TABLE 4	Common Eyelid Disorders	
DISEASE	**Si/Sx**	**Tx**
Chalazion	• Lipogranulomatous inflammation of internal meibomian sebaceous gland • Presents with swelling on conjunctival surface of eyelid	• Warm compresses, lid hygiene, usually self-limiting • Incision and currettage, send path specimen to rule out malignancy (sebaceous cell carcinoma), especially in recurrent lesions
Hordeolum (Stye)	• Infection of external sebaceous glands of Zeiss or Mol • Presents with tender red swelling at lid margin	• Warm compresses, can add topical antibiotics
Blepharitis	• Inflammation of eyelids & eyelashes due to infection *(Staph. Aureus)* or secondary to seborrhea • Presents with red, swollen eyelid margins, with dry flakes noted on lashes	• Wash lid margins daily with baby shampoo • Use warm compresses • Without Tx can extend along eyelid ulceration
Entropion	• Inturning of eyelid, commonly seen in aging, and post operative blepharoplasty or trachoma secondary to scarring • Lashes rub on cornea (trichiasis) and can cause scarring and possible loss of vision	• Surgical repair with horizontal lid tightening procedure or grafts to lengthen posterior portion of the eyelid
Ectropion	• Outward turning of eyelids, commonly seen in aging and post surgical scarring • Can also follow a cranial nerve VII palsy • Can lead to corneal ulceration from overly dry eye	• Surgical repair with horizontal lid tightening procedure and/or grafts to lengthen anterior portion of the eyelid

TABLE 4	*Continued*	
DISEASE	**Si/Sx**	**Tx**
Xanthelasma	• Painless flat yellow plaques occurring near inner canthi on eyelids	• Frequently associated with hyperlipidemias, rarely with Erdheim Chester disease—check for these • Surgical excision or CO_2 laser treatment
Basal cell carcinoma	• Pearly elevated nodule with central ulceration, lash loss; occasionally may be flat	• Complete surgical excision with micrographic technique or frozen section control

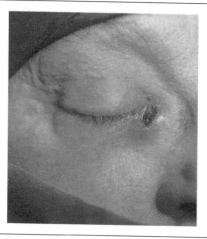

FIGURE 10   Dacrocystitis

    Hemophilus influenzae (children), *Pseudomonas,* or *S. pyogenes*

b. Caused by tear stasis secondary to nasolacrimal duct obstruction, trauma, lacrimal sac stones, sinus, and nasal abnormalities

c. Si/Sx = inflammation, erythema & tenderness of medial aspect of lower lid, purulent discharge may be noted or expressed from punctum, tearing

d. May see fistula or abscess formation of the lacrimal sac

e. Tx = warm soaks, systemic anti-*Staphylococcus*, and/or organism specific antibiotics

f. Dacrocystorhinostomy with stent placement may be needed for patients with repeated obstruction of tear duct

g. Orbital imaging if eye motility changes, proptosis, unresponsiveness to antibiotics

4. Dacroadenitis (tear gland inflammation)

a. Infection of lacrimal gland, usually caused by *Staphylococcus aureus, Streptococcus pneumoniae, Hemophilus influenzae*, or *S. pyogenes*

b. Si/Sx = inflammation, erythema, & tenderness of temporal aspect of upper lid (Lateral)

c. Tx = warm soaks, systemic anti-*Staphylococcus*, and/or organism specific antibiotics

C. Orbit

1. Orbital cellulitis (Table 5) (see Figures 11 and 12)

2. Graves (thyroid) ophthalmopathy

a. Immune mediated disease that attacks orbit and thyroid

b. Most common cause of unilateral and bilateral proptosis

c. Motility limitation secondary to infiltration of rectimuscles (inferior most common)

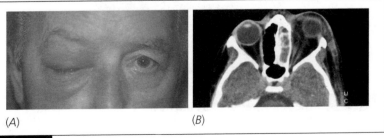

(A) (B)

FIGURE 11

(A) The clinical appearance of a patient with the right orbital cellulitis. (B) A CT scan showing a left opaque ethmoid sinus and subperiosteal orbital abscess.

TABLE 5	Orbital Cellulitis	
DIAGNOSIS	**Si/Sx's**	**TREATMENT**
Orbital Cell ulitis **Stages** 1. Preseptal cellulitis (periorbital) 2. Orbital cellulitis 3. Subperiosteal abscess 4. Orbital abscess 5. Cavernous sinus thrombosis	• Preseptal cellulitis—eyelid edema, erythema, warmth, and tenderness • Orbital cellulitis—proptosis, progressively impaired extraocular motility, pupil, and vision changes • Also seen as complication of paranasal sinus infection (ethmoids most commonly involved) • Can spread to cavernous sinus via <u>valveless</u> venous system leading to deadly thrombosis & meningitis	• ID, ophthalmology, and otolaryngology consult • CT scan of head and orbits with contrast to evaluate extent of disease • Treat emergently with IV antibiotics (Nafcillin & Unasyn®) to cover *Staph. Aureus* and paranasal sinus pathogens • If vision impaired or patient not improving on antibiotics. Surgery is indicated to drain sinuses or abscess

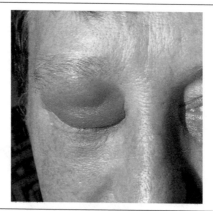

FIGURE 12 The Appearance of a Patient with Preseptal Cellulitis

d. Lid retraction

   1) Compressive optic neuropathy and corneal exposure main causes of vision loss

   2) Orbital decompression may be indicated for worsening Sx's.

3. Common orbital tumors

  a. Adult

    1) Cavernous hemangioma

      a) Most common adult tumor

      b) Large well-circumscribed vascular tumor

    2) Metastases

      a) Breast, lung, prostate most common

      b) 10% of orbital tumors

    3) Lymphoid tumors

      a) Older patients

      b) Spectrum from benign reactive lymphoid hyperplasia to lymphoma

      c) Orbital involvement alone—radiotherapy, if systemic, radiation and chemotherapy

    4) Fibrous histocytoma—mesenchymal tumor

    5) Mucocele—cystic mass of sinuses caused by duct obstruction, frontal and ethmoid sinuses most commonly involved

    6) Fibrous dysplasia—bony tumor

    7) Schwannoma

      a) Tumor of peripheral nerve

      b) Seen in neurofibromatosis

  b. Pediatric

    1) Capillary hemangioma (see Figure 13)

      a) Most common orbital tumor in children

      b) Vascular tumor

    2) Dermoid cyst (see Figure 14)

      a) Benign cystic mass with connective tissue and skin appendages (hair, sebaceous glands)

    3) Leukemia

      a) Myelogenous leukemia—chloroma

      b) Lymphocytic leukemia—can also produce orbital infiltration

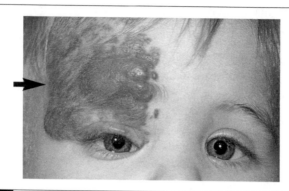

FIGURE 13 Capillary Hemangioma

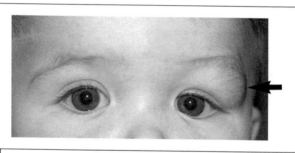

FIGURE 14 Dermoid Cyst of Left Superotemporal Orbit

4) Rhabdomyosarcoma

   a) Most common primary orbital malignancy in children

   b) Embryonal (most common), alveolar (worst prognosis), pleomorphic (best prognosis), botryoid

5) Lymphangioma

   a) Tumor of early childhood with large lymph channels

   b) Often have hemorrhage

6) Neuroblastoma

   a) Most common metastatic tumor in children

   b) Ecchymosis with proptosis

VIII. RETINOPATHY

A. Retina

1. Branch/central retinal artery occlusion (BRAO/CRAO)

   a. Retinal artery occlusion by emboli causes sudden, unilateral partial to complete painless loss of vision

   b. Pupil is sluggish to respond to direct light stimulation in CRAO

   c. BRAO caused by cholesterol, septic emboli, CRAO caused by embolus or thrombus

   d. Fovea will often contain a cherry-red spot in central retinal artery occlusion

   e. Associated with diabetes, hypertension, and carotid occlusive disease

   f. Patients have history of amaurosis fugax

2. Central/branch retinal vein occlusion (CRVO/BRVO)

   a. Caused by a thrombus

   b. Associated with diabetes, hypertension, hypercoagulable states, and coronary artery disease

   c. Physical finding = tortuous distended veins, retinal edema, numerous retinal hemorrhages

   d. Presents with painless, sudden loss of vision

3. Age-related macular degeneration (AMD)

   a. Progressive degeneration of the retinal pigment epithelium

   b. AMD causes gradual painless loss of visual acuity

   c. Dx by altered pigmentation in macula

   d. Severe vision loss secondary to choroidal neovascular membranes that leak and bleed patients tend to retain only peripheral vision

   e. Tx = laser to areas of membrane that leak, antioxidant vitamins

4. Retinitis pigmentosa (see Figure 15)

   a. Slowly progressive retinal degeneration that produces defect in night vision (often starts in young children) with ring-shaped scotoma (blind spot) that gradually increases in size to obscure vision

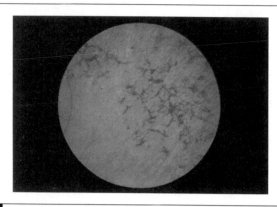

FIGURE 15 The Clinical Appearance of Peripheral Retina in Retinitis Pigmentosa

- b. Disease is hereditary with multiple modes of transmission (X-linked most severe)
- c. May be part of the Laurence-Moon-Biedl syndrome
- d. Some studies show vitamin A palmitate to be of benefit, no definitive therapy

5. Retinal detachment
   - a. Rhegmatogenous—secondary to a retinal tear or break
   - b. Traction—seen in diabetes, fibrovascular tissue pulling on retina, causing it to detach
   - c. Exudative—subretinal fluid from tumor or inflammation causing detachment of retina
   - d. Tx = surgery for large detachments, cryotherapy or laser for smaller breaks

6. Endophthalmitis
   - a. Intraocular infection
   - b. Can occur after trauma (*Bacillus cereus*), intraocular surgery (such as cataract—*S. aureus, Strep. spp.*)
   - c. Endogenous endophthalmitis can occur rarely—fungal (*Candida*)
   - d. Si/Sx include pain, photophobia, decreased vision, and red eye
   - e. Tx = surgery and intraocular antibiotics

IX. OCULAR MANIFESTATIONS OF SYSTEMIC DISEASE

A. Common Systemic Diseases

1. Diabetes

   a. Diabetic retinopathy

      1) Incidence increases with length of diabetes

      2) Leading cause of blindness in ages 25–40

         a) Background (nonproliferative)

            i) Dot and flame hemorrhages, microaneurysms & soft exudates (cotton-wool spots) on retina

            ii) Also see macular edema

            iii) Strict glucose control decreases the incidence of and progression to proliferative diabetic retinopathy

         b) Proliferative type

            i) More advanced dz, with neovascularization easily visible around optic nerve and retina

            ii) Can lead to vitreous hemorrhage, retinal detachment, and blindness

            iii) Tx is photocoagulation (laser ablation of neovascularization in the retina) and surgery

2. **Multiple Sclerosis (MS)**

   a. Retrobulbar neuritis

      1) Caused by idiopathic inflammation of the optic nerve, usually unilateral

      2) **Seen in multiple sclerosis, often is the initial sign**

      3) Si/Sx = rapid loss of vision & pain upon moving eye, spontaneously remitting within 2–8 wk, 70% of patients recover 20/20 vision

      4) Funduscopic exam is nonrevealing

      5) Tx = iv corticosteroids hasten final visual acuity and decreases incidence of MS for two years

3. **Hypertension**

   a. Can have retinal changes with acute or chronically elevated blood pressure

1) Arteriole narrowing
2) Copper wiring
3) Cotton-wool spots (nerve fiber layer infarcts)
4) Flame hemorrhages
5) Disc hyperemia and edema with dilated vessels in malignant hypertension

4. Ocular findings and associated medical conditions (Table 6) (see Figures 16 and 17 and Color Plate 5)

TABLE 6 Ocular Findings and Associated Medical Conditions	
Roth spots small hemorrhagic spots with central clearing in retina	Endocarditis
Copper wiring, flame hemorrhages, A-V nicking seen in subacute hypertension **cotton-wool spots** (soft exudates) seen in acute and chronic HTN	Hypertension and/or arteriosclerosis
Papilledema—disk hyperemia, blurring, & elevation	Increased Intracranial pressure
"Sea fan" neovascularization of retina	Sickle cell anemia
Cherry-red spot on macula	Tay-Sachs, Niemann-Pick disease, central retinal artery occlusion
Hollenhorst plaque	Yellow cholesterol emboli in retinal artery seen in atherosclerosis
Yellow eye (icterus)	Bilirubin staining of sclera (jaundice)
Yellow vision	Digoxin toxicity
Blue sclera	Osteogenesis imperfecta & Marfan's disease
Cataract	Causes congenital, diabetes (sorbitol precipitation in lens), galactosemia (galactitol precipitation in lens), Hurler's disease (defect in iduronidase mucopolysaccharide precipitation in lens)
Cancer/tumors Brown pigmented lesion on retina (Figure 17)	Malignant melanoma, most common intraocular tumor in adults (usually elevated), flat pigmented lesions are nevi

TABLE 6 *Continued*	
Eyelid ulceration with telangiectasias	Basal cell carcinoma most common eyelid malignancy
Lens dislocation	Occurs in homocystinuria, Marfan's & Alport' s syndromes. Lens **dislocates superiorly in Marfan's (mnemonic:** Marfan's patients are tall, their lenses dislocate upward), inferiorly in homocystinuria & variably in Alport's syndrome
Kayser-Fleischer ring	**Pathognomonic for Wilson's disease.** Finding is a ring of golden pigment on Descemet's membrane of the cornea
Argyll-Robertson pupil	**Pathognomonic for tertiary syphilis (neurosyphilis).** Pupils constrict with accommodation but do not constrict to direct light stimulation (pupils accommodate but do not react)

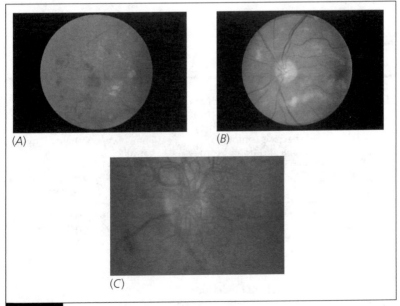

(A) (B) (C)

FIGURE 16 The Signs of Retinal Vascular Disease

(A) Hemorrhage and exudate; (B) cotton wool spots; (C) new vessels, here particularly florid arising at the disc. Note the yellowish nature and distinct margin to the exudates compared to the less distinct and white appearance of the cotton wool spot.

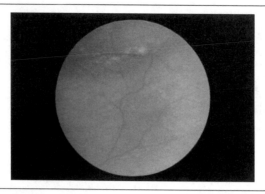

FIGURE 17 The Clinical Appearance of a Choroidal Melanoma

X. ORBITAL TRAUMA

A. Eye Related Trauma (Table 7)

TABLE 7	Eye Related Trauma	
DIAGNOSIS	**Si/Sx's**	**TREATMENT**
Chemical burns	• Alkali burns most damaging. Severe pain, erythema, conjunctival injection or blanching/necrosis complete opacification of cornea in severe cases	• Immediate irrigation of eye with normal saline and removal of particulate debris • Check vision and pH • Immediate ophthalmology consult • Complete history of events surrounding exposure and exam of eye, face, and airway
Eyelid laceration	• May be superficial or involve deeper structures such as levator muscle, tarsal plate, and orbital septum. Medial lacerations can include lacrimal system (canaliculus) • Penetrating foreign bodies must be ruled out as a cause of laceration	• Ophthalmology consult for repair of lid/lacrimal system

TABLE 7	*Continued*	
DIAGNOSIS	**Si/Sx's**	**TREATMENT**
Foreign body	• Pencils, glass, metal, wood, bullet • May cause corneal abrasion if hidden beneath eye lids • May be intraocular or intraorbital. CT scan is gold standard for imaging. (Never MRI, the magnet moves metallic object and may cause further damage) • Tear drop or odd shaped pupil occasionally seen with penetrating foreign bodies	• Ophthalmology consult • External examination of eye lids, orbital walls, conjunctiva, visual acuity, pupils, and extraocular movements. Slit-lamp examination of cornea with fluorescein dye • Eye shield prior to transport • Stabilize any objects protruding from orbit • Give IV broad spectrum antibiotics • Give antiemetics to control nausea and vomiting and prevent increased intraocular pressure • Tetanus prophylaxis • Glass and some metals are inert and are well tolerated. Wood must be removed immediately to prevent endophthalmitis
Ruptured globe (open globe injury)	• Full thickness corneal/corneoscleral/scleral laceration secondary to blunt or penetrating trauma	• **Urgent** surgical repair to close eye and IV antibiotics • Orbital imaging to look for intraocular foreign bodies BEWARE of sympathetic ophthalmia—a rare autoimmune uveitis that can affect the injured eye and then progresses to uninjured eye. Tx-enucleate any irreversibly injured globes
Retinal detachment	• Commonly associated with blunt trauma to eye • Presents with painless, dark vitreous floaters, flashes of light (photopsias), and blurry vision • Progresses to a curtain of blindness in vision as detachment worsens • Retinal tear or hole visualized in periphery • Wrinkles on retina seen in retinal detachment	• Ophthalmology consult for urgent surgical reattachment

TABLE 7	*Continued*	
DIAGNOSIS	**Si/Sx's**	**TREATMENT**
Hyphema	• Pain, blurriness blunt ocular trauma • Irregular pupil • Blood in anterior chamber of eye, fluid level noted	• Ophthalmology consult
Blowout fracture	• Thin bones of orbit "blow out" from increased intraorbital pressure. Most commonly orbital floor and medial wall • Enophthalmos, diplopia, and occasionally extraocular muscle entrapment, usually inferior rectus	• CT scan of orbit • Ophthalmology or • Otolaryngology consult
Traumatic optic neuropathy	• Caused by indirect trauma to optic nerve, direct trauma from compression by hematoma or bone fragments • Afferent pupillary defect (Marcus-Gunn pupil) • Vision loss	• Ophthalmology consult • Treatment controversial—observation vs. intravenous steroids (recent large study showed no benefit of steroids or decompression)
Retrobulbar Hemorrhage	• Can be seen with blunt trauma to eye and postoperatively after sinus surgery and blepharoplasty • Proptosis, resistance to retropulsion, increased intraocular pressure, decreased extraocular motility, and afferent pupillary defect	• Ophthalmology consult • Surgical lateral canthotomy and lateral tendon cantholysis to relieve pressure may be necessary

XI. EYE DRUGS

A. Eye Drops and Ointments (Table 8)

TABLE 8	Eye Drops and Ointments		
DRUG CLASS	**EXAMPLES**	**USE**	**SIDE EFFECTS**
Anesthetics	• Proparacaine hydrochloride • Tetracaine	• Decreases corneal sensation • Inhibiting corneal blink reflex and decreasing pain • Removal of foreign bodies and examination of injured cornea	• Repeated long-term use can lead to corneal ulceration, perforation • Can cause ocular allergic reaction
Steroids (topical)	• Prednisolone • Loteprednol • Rimexolone	• Iritis	• May potentiate a herpes simplex keratitis, bacterial or fungal infection if misdiagnosed • Cataracts and increased intraocular pressure seen in long-term use of steroid eye drops (steroid induced glaucoma) • Ophthalmologist directed use only

TABLE 8	*Continued*		
DRUG CLASS	**EXAMPLES**	**USE**	**SIDE EFFECTS**
Anticholinergics	• Short acting—Tropicamide, Cyclopentolate hydrochloride • Long acting—Scopolamine hydrobromide, Atropine sulfate	• Mydriatic and cycloplegic agents use to fully examine retina and facilitate refraction	• Rarely nausea, vomiting, and syncope • Acute angle closure glaucoma
Adrenergics	• Phenylephrine hydrochloride	• Mydriatic only, no cycloplegic effects	• Hypertension, and tachycardia at higher concentrations
Decongestants	• Naphazoline hydrochloride • Phenylephrine hydrochloride • Tetrahydrozaline hydrochloride	• Used to relieve red eye • Cause vaso-contriction of conjuctival vessels	• Rebound vasodilation and worsening red eye
Antibacterials	• Tobramycin • Ciprofloxacin • Sulfacetamide • Erythromycin	• Prophylactic or organism specific bacterial treatment • Under the direction of an ophthalmologist	• Allergic reactions • Tobramycin toxic to corneal epithelium
Antiviral	• Vidarabine • Trifluridine	• Herpes Simplex Virus	• Allergic reactions • Punctate keratopathy
Nonsteroidal anti-inflammatory	• Diclofenac • Ketorolac	• Ocular allergy	• Allergic reaction • Tachyphylaxis

TABLE 8	*Continued*		
DRUG CLASS	**EXAMPLES**	**USE**	**SIDE EFFECTS**
Glaucoma	• Betablockers, i.e., Timolol (nonselective), betaxolol (beta-1 selective)	• Decrease aqueous humor formation	• Systemic absorption can cause bronchospasm, bradycardia, and hypotension
	• **Parasympatho-mimetics, i.e., Pilocarpine**	• Increase outflow	• Lacrimation, salivation, nausea, vomiting, and headache
	• Sympathomime-tic Epinephrine (beta agonist), iopidine (alpha agonist)	• Increase outflow (beta agonist), decrease aqueous production (alpha agonist)	• Hypertension, head ache, cardiac arrhythmias (iopidine causes allergic reaction)
	• Carbonic anhydrase inhibitors (Acetazolamide)	• Decrease aqueous formation	• Allergic reactions (sulfa base), nausea, vomiting, tingling of hands/feet. Avoid in patients with sickle cell trait or anemia, causes acidosis which increases sickling
Dry eye	Artificial tears	Ophthalmic lubricant	Allergic reaction to preservatives

PART TWO

OTORHINOLARYNGOLOGY
(ENT—EAR, NOSE, and THROAT)

XII. EMBRYOLOGY AND CONGENITAL DISORDERS

A. Basic Embryology

1. Branchial derivatives (Table 9)

TABLE 9	**Branchial Derivatives**			
LEVEL	**GROOVE (ECTODERM)**	**ARCH (MESODERM)**	**POUCH (ENDODERM)**	**ARTERY**
1	Pinna External auditory meatus	• Meckel's cartilage • Mandible, malleus, incus • Masticator muscles, mylohyoid, anterior belly of digastric, tensor tympani, tensor veli palatini • Parotid gland • Submandibular gland • CN V$_3$	• Eustachian tube • Middle ear cavity	• Maxillary
2		• Reichert's cartilage • Styloid process, stapes suprastructure • Stapedius muscle, anterior tongue muscles, muscles of facial expression, stylohyoid, posterior belly of digastric • CN VII	• Palatine tonsil	• Stapedial & hyoid
3		• Posterior tongue muscles, stylopharyngeus • CN IX	• Vallecular recess • Thymus • Inferior parathyroids	• Common carotid • Proximal internal carotid
4		• Thyroid cartilage • Cricothyroid muscle • CN X, superior laryngeal nerve	• Superior parathyroids	• Left aortic arch • Right subclavian

TABLE 9	*Continued*			
LEVEL	GROOVE (ECTODERM)	ARCH (MESODERM)	POUCH (ENDODERM)	ARTERY
5			• Parafollicular cells	
6		• Cricoid & arytenoid cartilage • Larynx muscles • CN X, inferior laryngeal nerve	• Laryngeal ventricle	• Proximal pulmonary artery • Ductus arteriosus

Note: Otic vesicle is the surface ectoderm derived embryonic structure that forms inner ear. It divides into a utricular portion-utricle, semicircular canals, and endolymphatic duct, and a saccular portion-saccule, and cochlear duct.

B. Congenital Disorders

1. Cleft lip

    a. Can occur unilaterally or bilaterally

    b. Unilateral cleft lip is the most common malformation of the head & neck

    c. Caused by failure of fusion of maxillary prominences

    d. Multifactorial causes, associated with Van der Woude syndrome, and in utero teratogens

    e. Commonly surgically repaired by age 1–3 months or

    f. Rule of 10's—10 wk—10 lb—Hgb of 10 needed for repair

2. Cleft palate

    a. Can be anterior or posterior (determined by position relative to incisive foramen)

    b. Anterior cleft palate (primary clefting) due to failure of palatine shelves to fuse with primary palate. Occurs anterior to incisive foramen

    c. Posterior cleft palate (secondary clefting) due to failure of palatine shelves to fuse with nasal septum. Occurs posterior to incisive foramen

    d. Tx = surgical repair of palate at age 18–24 months after eruption of the first molars

    e. These patients also commonly require pressure equalization tubes for eustachian tube dysfunction to prevent middle ear disease

    f. Feeding difficulties and velopharyngeal insufficiency—hypernasal speech and nasal regurgitation are commonly seen in these patients

3. Choanal atresia

    a. Lack of orifice at choanae connecting nares & nasopharynx. Can be due to membranous obstruction vs. a bony obstruction

    b. **Classic presentation = cyanotic newborn whose hypoxia abates during crying** (babies are obligate nasal breathers, but crying forces mouth breathing)

    c. Can be seen in CHARGE associations—coloboma, heart defects, Atresia of choanae, retardation, genital defects, ear disorders, or deafness

    d. Dx = Inability to pass a suction catheter or fiberoptic scope transnasally or CT scan makes the diagnosis

    e. Tx = surgical dilation or resection

4. Kartagener's syndrome

    a. Immotile cilia syndrome due to absence of dynein arms

    b. Patients are infertile (sperm do not work without dynein), with ↓ olfaction, sinusitis, bronchiectasis, & situs inversus

    c. Frequent respiratory infections due to lack of mucociliary escalator

5. Osler-Weber-Rendu syndrome (hereditary hemorrhagic telangiectasia) (see Figure 18 and Color Plate 6)

    a. Autosomal dominant disorder of diffuse telangiectasias on lips, skin & mucous membranes, & internal organs

    b. Sx = severe nosebleed, hemoptysis, massive GI bleeds

    c. Dx = unexplained GI bleeds + typical red/violet telangiectasias

    d. Tx = epistaxis is supportive, e.g., blood transfusions, occasionally surgical removal of nasal mucosa with skin graft

6. Cystic fibrosis

    a. Can present with chronic & severe pansinusitis in children (*Pseudomonas spp.*)

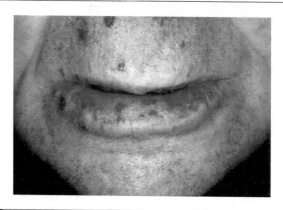

FIGURE 18 The Lesions of Hereditary Telangectasia

b. Dx = sweat chloride test in older children. In infants & toddlers (up to 2 yr) sweat test is unreliable, genetic screening indicated

c. Tx = supportive, pancreatic enzymes, and sinus surgery

d. Note: Classic sign on CT scans of the sinuses (coronal view) —medial bowing of the medial maxillary walls from the maxillary sinus polyposis. These patients can live a lot longer than before, but most require multiple sinus operations

7. Hutchinson's teeth

a. Notching of the permanent upper 2 incisors

b. **Pathognomonic for congenital syphilis**

c. **Part of Hutchinson's triad = notched teeth, keratitis, & deafness**

8. Macroglossia

a. Congenitally enlarged tongue

b. Occurs in cretinism, Down's syndrome, and gigantism

c. Can also be acquired in amyloidosis, acromegaly, and hypothyroidism

d. This is different from glossitis (redness & swelling, with burning sensation) seen in vitamin B deficiencies

9. First arch syndromes

a. Treacher Collins—mandibulofascial dyostosis—microtia (external ear hypoplasia), underdeveloped zygomatic arches, malar hypoplasia, down-turned palpebral fissures, colobomas of lower eyelids

   b. Pierre-Robin sequence—micrognathia (small mandible), glossoptosis (posteriorly placed tongue), and cleft palate

10. DiGeorge's syndrome

   a. 3rd and 4th pharyngeal pouch syndrome

   b. Thymic hypoplasia or aplasia—T-cell immunodeficiency, parathyroid hypoplasia-calcium disregulation, heart defects, hypertelorism (widely spaced eyes), and middle ear defects

11. Craniosynostosis

   a. Premature closure of calvarial sutures (coronal, lamboid, metopic, and sagittal)

   b. Causes a deformity of skull and its contents

   c. Tx = surgery

12. Congenital midline nasal masses

   a. Dermoid—composed of ectoderm and mesoderm and occurs along embryonic fusion lines (midline)

   b. Encephalocele—herniated glial tissue that maintains communication with CSF

      1) Caused by a persistence of Fonticularis Frontalis Encephalocele tract

      2) + Furstenburg sign—(mass enlarges with straining or crying)

   c. Glioma—collection of ectodermal neural tissue not usually connected to CSF

13. Histiocytosis X

   a. Proliferation of histiocytic cells resembling Langerhans skin cells

   b. Can present with epistaxis or nasal mass

   c. Three common variants

      1) Letterer-Siwe disease

         a) Acute, aggressive, disseminated variant, usually fatal in infants

         b) Si/Sx = hepatosplenomegaly, lymphadenopathy, pancytopenia, lung involvement, recurrent infections

    2) Hand-Schuller-Christian

        a) Chronic progressive variant, presents prior to 5 yr old

        b) **Classic triad = skull lesions, diabetes insipidus, exophthalmus**

    3) Eosinophilic granuloma

        a) Extraskeletal involvement generally limited to lung

        b) Has the best Px, rarely fatal, sometimes spontaneously regresses

14. Down's syndrome

    a. **Invariably caused by trisomy 21, ↑ risk if maternal age >35 yr**

    b. Si/Sx → cardiac septal defects, psychomotor retardation, classic Down's facies, ↑ risk of leukemia, premature Alzheimer's dz

    c. Down's facies = flattened occiput (brachycephaly), **epicanthal folds, up-slanted palpebral fissures, speckled irises (Brushfield spots)**, protruding tongue, small ears, redundant skin at posterior neck, **hypotonia, simian crease in palms (50%)**, and atlantoaxial laxity.

    d. Px = typically death in 30–40s

15. Turner's syndrome

    a. **No.1 cause of 1° amenorrhea,** due to XO genotype

    b. Si/Sx = newborns have ↑ skin at dorsum of neck (**neck webbing**), lymphedema in hands & feet, as develop → short stature, ptosis, **coarctation of aorta, amenorrhea but uterus is present**, juvenile external genitalia, bleeding due to GI telangiectasias, no mental retardation

    c. Tx = hormone replacement to allow 2° sex characteristics to develop

16. Fragile X syndrome

    a. X-linked dominant trinucleotide repeat expansion disorder

    b. **No. 1 cause of mental retardation in boys**

    c. Si/Sx = long face, prominent jaw, large ears, enlarged testes (postpubertal), developmental delay, mental retardation

    d. Tx = none

17. Arnold-Chiari malformation

    a. Congenital disorder

    b. Si/Sx = caudally displaced cerebellum, elongated medulla passing into foramen magnum, flat skull base, hydrocephalus, meningomyelocele, aqueductal stenosis, vocal cord paralysis

    c. Px = death as neonate or toddler

18. Fetal alcohol syndrome

    a. Seen in children born to alcoholic mothers

    b. Si/Sx = characterized by facial abnormalities & developmental defects (mental & growth retardation), **smooth filtrum of lip,** microcephaly, atrial septal defect

    c. Tx = prevention

19. Achondroplasia

    a. Very common cause of dwarfism, autosomal dominant

    b. Early sealing off between epiphysis & metaphysis, causes shortening/thickening of bones

    c. Sx = leg bowing, hearing loss, sciatica, infantile hydrocephalus

    d. Patients can live normal lifespans

20. Fibrous dysplasia

    a. Idiopathic replacement of bone with fibrous tissue, three types: a) monostotic, b) polystotic, c) McCune-Albright's

        1) Monostotic pts are often aSx, but can suffer spontaneous fractures

        2) Polystotic are associated with severe skeletal deformity

        3) McCune-Albright's syndrome

            a) Caused by G-protein abnormality resulting in hyperparathyroidism, hyperadrenalism, & acromegaly

            b) **Triad = polystotic fibrous dysplasia, precocious puberty, café-au-lait spots**

21. Marfan's disease

    a. Defect in the fibrillin gene causes connective tissue abnormality

    b. Tall, thin body habitus, digits are characteristically long & slender

    c. Patients have both pectus excavatum & scoliosis

TABLE 10	The TORCHS
DISEASE	**CHARACTERISTICS**
Toxoplasmosis	• Acquired in mothers via ingestion of poorly cooked meat or through contact with cat feces • Carriers common (10–30%) in population, only causes neonatal dz if acquired during pregnancy (1%) • One third of women who acquire during pregnancy transmit infection to fetus, & one third of fetuses are clinically affected • Sequelae = intracerebral calcifications, hydrocephalus, chorioretinitis, microcephaly, severe mental retardation, epilepsy, intrauterine growth retardation (IUGR), hepatosplenomegaly • Screening is useless since acquisition prior to infection is common & clinically irrelevant • Pregnant women should be told to avoid undercooked meat, wash hands after handling cat, do not change litter box • If fetal infection established → Utz to determine major anomalies & provide counseling
Rubella	• First trimester maternal Rubella infxn → 80% chance of fetal transmission • Second trimester → 50% chance of transmission to fetus, third trimester → 5% • Si/Sx of fetus = intrauterine growth retardation, cataracts, glaucoma, chorioretinitis, patent ductus arteriosus, pulmonary stenosis, atrial or ventricular septal defect, myocarditis, microcephaly, **hearing loss, "blueberry muffin rash,"** mental retardation • Dx confirmed with IgM Rubella Ab in neonate's serum, or viral culture • Tx = prevention by universal immunization of all children against Rubella, there is no effective therapy for active infection
Cytomegalovirus (CMV)	• No. 1 congenital infection, affecting 1% of births • Transmitted through bodily fluids/secretions, infection often asymptomatic • 1° seroconversion during pregnancy → ↑ risk of severely affected infant, but congenital infection can occur if mother reinfected during pregnancy • About 1% risk of transplacental transmission of infection, about 10% of infected infants manifest congenital defects of varying severity • Congenital defects = microcephaly, intracranial calcifications, severe mental retardation, chorioretinitis, IUGR • 10–15% of asymptomatic but exposed infants will develop later neurologic sequelae

TABLE 10 *Continued*	
DISEASE	**CHARACTERISTICS**
Herpes simplex virus	• **C-section delivery for pregnant women with active herpes** • Vaginal →50% chance that the baby will acquire the infection & is associated with significant morbidity & morality • Si/Sx = vesicles, seizures, respiratory distress, can cause pneumonia, meningitis, encephalitis →impaired neurologic development after resolution • Tx = acyclovir (markedly decreases mortality)
Syphilis	• Transmission from infected mother to infant during pregnancy nearly 100%, **occurs after the first trimester in the vast majority of cases** • Fetal/perinatal deaths in 40% of affected infants • Early manifestations in first 2 years, later manifestations in next 2 decades • Si/Sx of early dz = jaundice, ↑ liver function tests, hepatosplenomegaly, hemolytic anemia, rash followed by desquamation of hands & feet, wart-like lesions of mucous membranes, **blood-tinged nasal secretions (snuffles), diffuse osteochondritis, saddle nose (2° to syphilitic rhinitis)** • Si/Sx of late dz = **Hutchinson teeth** (notching of permanent upper 2 incisors), mulberry molars (both at 6 yr), bone thickening (frontal bossing), **anterior bowing of tibia (saber shins)** • Dx = RPR/VDRL & FTA serologies in mother with clinical findings in infant • Tx = procaine penicillin G for 10–14 days

    d. Cardiac involvement includes progressive aortic valve dilation leading to regurgitation, aortic dissection, & mitral valve prolapse

    e. **Hallmark is joint laxity, also optic lens dislocations & blue sclera**—lens dislocation upward in Marfan's as opposed to downward in homocystinuria

XIII. HEADACHE

A. Signs/Symptoms & Differential Diagnosis

1. Summary of headaches (Table 11)

TABLE 11	Summary of Headaches	
TYPE	**EPIDEMIOLOGY**	**CHARACTERISTICS**
Tension	Usually after age 20 (rarely >age 50)	• Most common headache type • **Bilateral, band-like, dull in quality** • Worse with stress; not aggravated by activity • Chronic HA associated with depression
Cluster	**Male:female = 6:1** Mean age 30 yr	• **Unilateral**, stabbing peri/retro-orbital pain, lasting 15 min to 3 hr • Seasonal attacks occur in series (6x/day) lasting weeks, followed by months of remission • **Associated with ipsilateral lacrimation (85%), ptosis, nasal congestion & rhinorrhea** • Often occurs within 90 min of onset of sleep
Migraine	80% have positive Family Hx **Female:male = 3:1**	• Classically, HA is **unilateral (60%)** with **aura (only 15%)**; pt looks for quiet place to rest • Visual aura: **scotoma** (blind spots), **teichopsia** (jagged zigzag lines), **photopsias** (shimmering lights), or **rhodopsins** (colors) • Accompanied by **nausea & photophobia**, vertigo • Triggered by stress, odors, certain foods, alcohol, menstruation, or sleep deprivation
Temporal arteritis (Giant cell)	**Female:male = 2:1** Age >50	• **Unilateral temporal** headache • **Associated with jaw claudication, temporal artery tenderness with palpation, ESR ≥50** • 50% also have polymyalgia rheumatica • If not treated leads to optic neuritis & **blindness** • Screen by ESR; Dx with temporal artery Bx
Trigeminal neuralgia	Peak age at 60 or secondary to viral infection or trauma	• Episodic, severe pain shooting from side of mouth to ipsilateral ear, eye, or nose
Withdrawal headache		• Common cause of frequent headaches • Can be withdrawal from various drugs
SAH*		• Head trauma is most common cause • Spontaneous: usually berry aneurysm rupture • Classically the "worst headache of my life"

*Subarachnoid hemorrhage.

B. Dx Is Made by Clinical History & Physical Except:

1. **Temporal arteritis Dx requires temporal artery biopsy**

2. **Trigeminal neuralgia** a diagnosis of exclusion **Dx requires head CT or MRI** to rule out sinusitis, cerebellopontine angle neoplasm, multiple sclerosis, herpes zoster

3. **Subarachnoid hemorrhage requires** confirmation by CT scan or lumbar puncture to detect CSF xanthochromia (can be detected 6 hr after onset of HA)

4. Suspect intracranial lesion causing headache in **pts >50 or pts with headaches immediately upon waking up**

5. Suspect ↑ ICP in pts awakened in middle of night by headache, who have projectile vomiting, or focal neural deficits; obtain head CT

C. Treatment of Headache (Table 12)

TABLE 12	Treatment of Headaches
HEADACHE	**TREATMENT**
Tension	• Acutely NSAIDs or Midrin® • Prophylaxis with antidepressants or β-blockers
Cluster	• Acutely 100% O_2, sumatriptan* or dihydroergotamine • Prophylaxis with verapamil, lithium, methysergide,** or ergotamine
Migraine	• Acutely sumatriptan,* dihydroergotamine, methysergide,** NSAIDs, antiemetics
Temporal arteritis	• Prophylaxis with β-**blockers** (first line) or calcium blockers
Trigeminal neuralgia	• High-dose prednisone or cytotoxic drug to prevent blindness • Carbamazepine (first line) or phenytoin, clonazepam, valproic acid
Withdrawal	• NSAIDs
SAH	• Immediate neurosurgical evaluation & nimodipine to reduce incidence of postrupture vasospasm & ischemia

*Sumatriptan contraindicated with known coronary dz or ergot drugs taken within 24 hr.
** Beware of fibrosis of retroperitoneum, pleura and cardiac valves. A classic side effect of long-term use.

XIV. EARS

A. Otitis Externa (OE)

1. Most commonly caused by aggressive cleaning of ears with cotton swabs or "swimmer's ear" seen in those who frequently have excessive moisture in their ears

   a. Cerumen is composed of antibacterial lysozymes that protect ears from infection

2. Si/Sx = pain, **pruritis, and ottorhea. External auditory canal may appear swollen and pulling on pinna or pushing on tragus causes pain or tenderness**

3. *Pseudomonas* and *S. aureus* are usual cause, can be chronic in pts with seborrhea, and psoriasis

4. Tx = usually antibiotic ear drops and the prevention of water entering ear. Severe swelling of canal may require placement of a wick to ensure patency of external auditory canal and facilitate antibiotic delivery into canal (wick = gauze or small sponge)

5. **Otomycosis (Fungal OE)**

   a. Common in warm humid climates, frequent hair washing, immunosuppressed patients, and chronic OE treated with longterm **steroid** drops

   b. Common organisms *Aspergillus niger, Aspergillus albicans*, and *Candida albicans*

   c. Si/Sx = extremely itchy ear, drainage, black or white spots noted along canal wall and within cerumen

   d. Tx = Mycolog (nystatin and triamcinolone) ointment into ear canal. Careful suctioning and cleaning of canal with frequent follow-up

6. **Ramsay Hunt syndrome** (herpes zoster otiticus)

   a. Herpes infection of geniculate ganglia (CN VII)

   b. Si/Sx = painful vesicles in external auditory meatus

   c. Patients may develop facial paralysis

   d. Tx = urgent acyclovir to prevent progression to meningitis

7. **Malignant otitis externa**—a progressive destructive osteomyelitis of temporal bone more common in diabetics and immunosuppressed

   a. Green drainage from ear, severe mastoid tenderness

b. If suspected, get Technitium and gallium scan of temporal bone to rule out osteomyelitis or CT scan

c. Tx = IV anti-*Pseudomonas* antibiotics, daily suctioning and local ear care. Those who are progressing despite this, or have intracranial involvement may go on to have surgical debridement

8. **Gradenigo syndrome**—osteomeylitis of petrous apex bone, causing ipsilateral ottorhea, eye pain, abducens paralysis (CN VI), diplopia

B. Otitis Media (OM)

1. Defined as inflammation of middle ear space

a. Dx = fever, erythema of tympanic membrane (TM), bulging of the pars flaccida portion of the TM, opacity of the TM, otalgia

b. Effusions can also be seen as meniscus of fluid behind the TM indicative of poor pressure equalization by eustachian tubes

c. Otitis media with effusion common in young children due to their eustachian tubes being smaller & more horizontal, making drainage and pressure equalization more difficult

d. Pathogens = *S. pneumoniae, Hemophilus influenzae, Moraxella catarrhalis*

e. Also commonly caused by viral pathogens

f. Tx = amoxicillin or azithromycin (first line), augmented penicillins or bactrim (second line)

g. If chronic effusions or repeated infections are present, surgical placement of pressure equalization (PE) tubes may be indicated

h. Note: Adults with unilateral serous effusion need to have a nasopharyngeal mass ruled out

i. Complication of otitis media and mastoiditis (see Figure 19 and Color Plate 7)

1) Intracranial-subdural abscess, epidural abscess, temporal lobe abscess, lateral sinus thrombosis, meningitis

2) Extracranial-facial paralysis, labrynthitis, and sub-periosteal abscess

CHRONIC OTITIS MEDIA

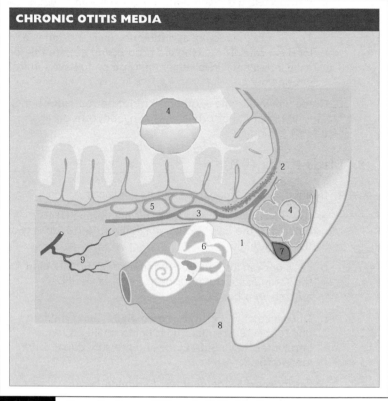

FIGURE 19 | **Complications of Chronic Otitis Media**

1) Acute mastoiditis. 2) Meningitis. 3) Extradural abscess. 4) Brain abscess (temporal lobe and cerebellum). 5) Subdural abscess. 6) Labyrinthitis. 7) Lateral sinus thrombosis. 8) Facial nerve paralysis. 9) Petrositis.

  3) Subperiosteal abscess

   a) Bezold's abscess = infection penetrates tip of mastoid and pus travels along sternocleidomastoid muscle and forms an abscess in posterior triangle of neck

   b) Postauricular abscess = most common subperiosteal abscess. Abscess posterior to auricle displacing ear

  4) ENT consult for surgical drainage and IV antibiotics

2. Bullous myringitis

 a. Associated with *Mycoplasma* infection

      b. Presents with large blebs on tympanic membrane

      c. Tx = erythromycin

  3. Unilateral serous otitis media

      a. Presents in adults, caused by nasopharyngeal masses obstructing the eustachian tube

      b. Dx = MRI of head, endoscopic visualization, and bx

C. Masses

  1. Cholesteatoma

      a. Most common growth in middle ear

      b. Can be congenital or acquired. Appearing as a retraction pocket in tympanic membrane and occasionally an actual mass is seen behind tympanic membrane

      c. It is an epithelial cyst that contains desquamated keratin and is often associated with inflammation (typically presents after chronic otitis media episodes)

      d. *Pseudomonas* can infect the keratin debris

      e. If left untreated, it can produce hearing loss. Can destroy bone & cause deafness & unilateral facial nerve paralysis. See chronic otitis media complications

      f. Tx = surgical removal

  2. Glomus tumors (paragangliomas)

      a. Most common true neoplasm of middle ear (glomus tympanicum)

      b. More common in high altitudes. Present with red pulsating mass behind tympanic membrane, conductive hearing loss, and pulsatile tinnitus

      c. Usually benign, can be associated with catecholamine release. Order urine VMA vanillyl mandelic acid and circulating catecholamines. R/o adrenal phechromocytoma

      d. Tx = surgery, radiation, or observation

3. Cholesterol granuloma (cyst)

   a. **Diagnostic dark bluish color of tympanic membrane without any prior trauma** (idiopathic hemotympanum)

   b. Bluish color due to foreign body reaction to cholesterol crystals from breakdown of blood

   c. Cystic structure may expand producing symptoms from mass effect

D. Relapsing Polychondritis

1. Autoimmune systemic disorder characterized by recurrent episodes of cartilage inflammation

2. Can involve any type of cartilage—ear, nose, and larynx

3. Diagnoses made on history of relapsing episodes of affected areas. Tissue biopsy not usually helpful

4. Associated with vasculitis, Lupus, and Sjogrens, Behcets

5. Commonly mistaken for **acute gout flare**, or infectious perichondritis, which presents in a similar fashion but commonly associated with insect bite

6. Sx = sudden bright red external ear pain and inflammation sparing lobule (no cartilage in lobule). Typically febrile and bilateral/occasionally hoarseness, conductive hearing loss, eye inflammation, nasal swelling

7. Tx = steroids

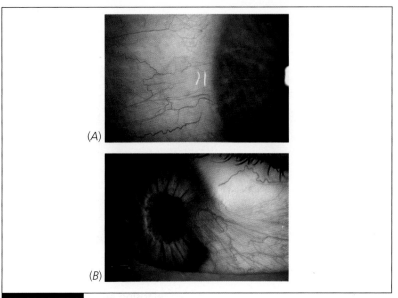

COLOR PLATE 1

The clinical appearance of (A) a pingueculum; (B) a pterygium.

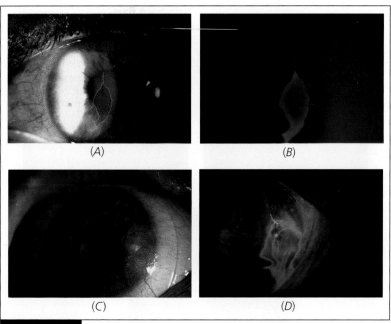

COLOR PLATE 2

(A) A corneal abrasion (the corneal epithelial layer has been damaged).
(B) Fluorescein uniformly stains the area of damage. (C) A perforated cornea
leaking aqueous (the leak is protected here with a soft contact lens).
(D) The fluorescein fluoresces as it is diluted by the leaking aqueous.

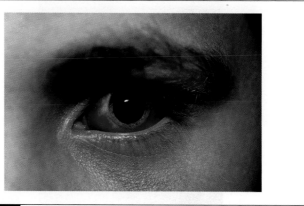

COLOR PLATE 3 A Subconjunctival Hemorrhage

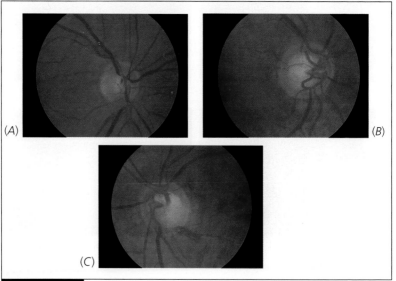

(A)

(B)

(C)

COLOR PLATE 4

Comparison of (A) a normal optic disc; (B) glaucomatous optic disc; (C) a disc hemorrhage is a feature of patients with low-tension glaucoma.

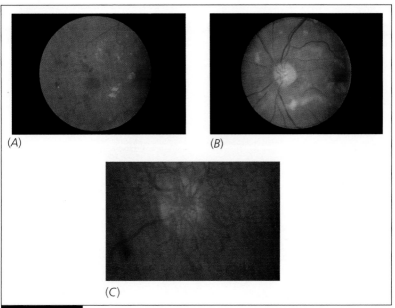

(A)　　　　　　　　　　(B)

(C)

COLOR PLATE 5　The Signs of Retinal Vascular Disease

(A) Hemorrhage and exudate; (B) cotton wool spots; (C) new vessels, here particularly florid arising at the disc. Note the yellowish nature and distinct margin to the exudates compared to the less distinct and white appearance of the cotton wool spot.

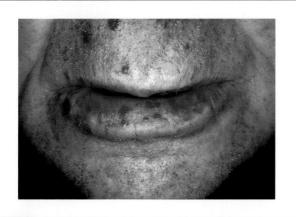

COLOR PLATE 6　The Lesions of Hereditary Telangectasia

CHRONIC OTITIS MEDIA

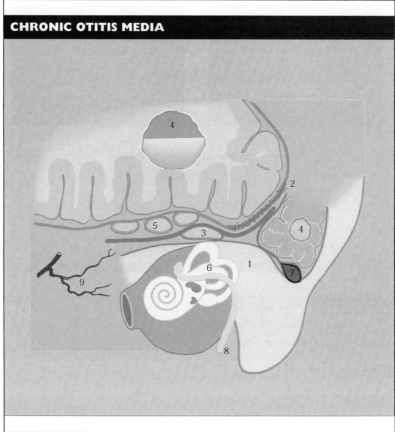

COLOR PLATE 7   **Complications of Chronic Otitis Media**

1) Acute mastoiditis. 2) Meningitis. 3) Extradural abscess. 4) Brain abscess (temporal lobe and cerebellum). 5) Subdural abscess. 6) Labyrinthitis. 7) Lateral sinus thrombosis. 8) Facial nerve paralysis. 9) Petrositis.

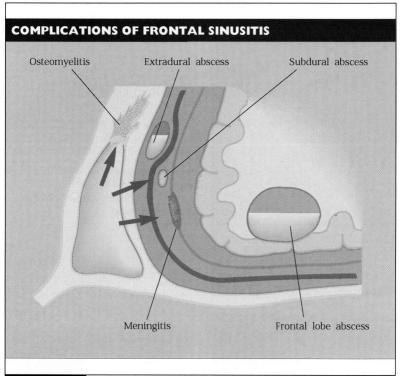

COLOR PLATE 8   **Complications of Frontal Sinusitis**

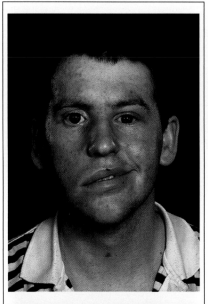

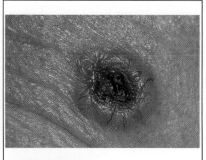

COLOR PLATE 10 Classic
Crateriform Basal Cell Carcinoma.
Ulcerating Nodule

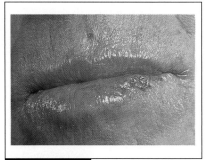

COLOR PLATE 11 Squamous Cell
Carcinoma of the Lip (Early Ulcer)

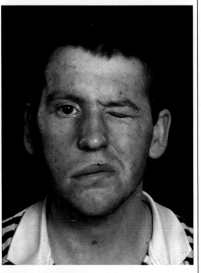

COLOR PLATE 9 Post-traumatic
Right Facial Palsy

*Shown at rest and on attempted eye
closure.*

E. ENT and Gout

1. **Monoarticular arthritis** due to urate crystal deposits in joints and on cartilage

2. Si/Sx of gout = painful monoarticular arthritis affecting distal joints (often first metatarsophalangeal joint, where disease is called **"podagra"**), **overlying skin erythema can mimic cellulitis or auricular perichondritis**

3. Dx

   a. Often based on clinical triad of monoarticular arthritis, hyperuricemia, ⊕ response to colchicine

   b. To differentiate from pseudogout, needle tap with analysis of crystals in joint must be performed

   c. **Beware—an acute attack can be precipitated by a sudden fall in serum urate levels, so pts do not always have a high urate level during an acute attack**

4. Acute Tx = colchicine (inhibits neutrophil inflammatory response to urate crystals) & NSAIDs (not aspirin!)

5. Pseudogout

   a. Caused by calcium pyrophosphate dihydrate (CPPD) crystal deposition in joints & articular cartilage (chondrocalcinosis)

   b. Mimics gout very closely, seen in persons age 60 or older, often affects larger, more proximal joints

   c. Can be 1° or 2° to metabolic dz (hyperparathyroidism, Wilson's dz, diabetes, hemochromatosis)

   d. Dx → microscopic analysis of joint aspirate

   e. Tx = colchicine & NSAIDs

6. Microscopy

   a. Gout → needle-like negatively birefringent crystals

   b. "P" seudogout → "P"ositively birefringent crystals

F. Hearing Loss

1. **Sensorineural hearing loss**

   a. Secondary to sensory damage of the organ of corti in the cochlea or retrocochlear damage such as from an acoustic neuroma or other CN VIII nerve damage

   b. May be of sudden onset, but most often slowly progressive

      1) Presbycusis—gradual loss of high frequency hearing as a person ages

      2) Sudden hearing loss is an emergency and immediate ENT referral should be made for appropriate diagnosis and treatment

      3) Bilateral hearing loss commonly associated with drugs, i.e., loop diuretics, aminoglycosides, salicylates, and cisplatin

   c. Potential causes include idiopathic, acoustic neuroma, congenital genetic, autoimmune, infection, inheritance, trauma, or toxins affecting nerve or cochlea

   d. Alport's syndrome

      1) Autoimmune sensorineural hearing loss, lens dislocation, hematuria

      2) Most likely X-linked dominant inheritance

      3) Thinning glomerular basement membrane and glomerulonephritis resulting in hematuria

e. Congenital—refers to sensorineural hearing loss at birth, does not specify etiology

   1) Etiologies include genetic, infectious, i.e., exposure of fetus to CMV, rubella or syphilis in utero

   2) Tx = hearing aids, cochlear implants and steroids commonly used. ENT consult recommended

2. Conductive hearing loss

   a. Due to malfunction of conduction pathway such as damage or obstruction affecting middle ear or external ear

   b. Examples include otitis media, excess cerumen, otosclerosis, cholesteatoma, or perforated tympanic membrane

   c. Mixed hearing loss (sensorineural and conductive) can be seen in chronic middle ear infection

   d. Usually correctable with surgery or appropriate treatment

   e. Patients often benefit from hearing aids

3. Diagnostic hearing tests

   a. Weber's test

      1) Vibrating tuning fork (512 Hz) is placed midline on top of head

      2) Lateralization of hearing to one ear more than the other indicates ipsilateral conductive loss or contralateral sensorineural loss

   b. Rinne's test (comparison of air conduction to bone conduction)

      1) Vibrating tuning fork (512 Hz) placed next to ear, then when no longer heard placed against mastoid process until no longer heard

      2) Normally air conduction should persist twice as long as bone conduction

3) Positive Rinne = air conduction heard longer and louder than bone conduction (this is the normal finding)

4) Negative Rinne = bone conduction is heard longer than air conduction, indicating a conductive hearing loss in that ear

c. Audiogram

1) A graphic representation of a patient's pure-tone responses to various auditory frequency stimuli (250–8000 Hz)

2) Should be obtained in all patients with changes in hearing or new onset tinnitus or vertigo

3) Hearing is considered normal when hearing thresholds are less than 20 decibels

4) Air-bone gaps (a difference between the air conduction and the bone conduction lines) exist when there is a conductive hearing loss

5) Asymmetric hearing loss may be indicative of an acoustic neuroma and further testing is needed with auditory brain response measurements and/or MRI with gadolinium

4. Tinnitus (ringing in the ears)

a. Objective (heard by observer) or subjective (heard only by patient)

b. Causes = foreign body in external canal, pulsating vascular tumors, medications (aspirin), and hearing loss (neuronal damage)

XV. DIZZY PATIENT (VERTIGO)

A. Vertigo (Dizzy Patient)

1. Vertigo—a sensation of rotation or movement of one's self or one's surroundings

2. Dizziness—a disturbed sense of relationship to space, a feeling of unsteadiness or lightheadedness

3. **Unilateral peripheral lesions**—affect labyrinth or cranial nerve VIII

a. Pts demonstrate nystagmus based on the location of the disease within the labyrinth. Peripheral nystagmus may be suppressed with fixation of vision. Frenzl glasses commonly used to prevent fixation and facilitate identification of nystagmus

b. May also have tinnitus or hearing loss

4. **Bilateral peripheral lesions**—can be caused by toxic substances such as gentamicin or by Ménière's disease

a. Both are commonly bilateral and have absence of nystagmus if both sides are affected equally

5. **Central lesions**—affect brain or cerebellum

a. Vertical nystagmus. Not suppressed by fixation

b. Depends on cause. Rule out ischemic brain injury

c. ENT or neurolgy consult

6. **Tx** = avoid antivertigo medications if possible in order to encourage the body to adapt. If symptoms are severe may treat with benzodiazepines or meclizine. Physical therapy may aid in the rehabilitation of these patients

TABLE 13	Dizzy Patient	
DISEASE	**CHARACTERISTICS**	**TREATMENT**
Benign paroxysmal positional vertigo (BPPV)	Sudden, episodic vertigo with head movement lasting for seconds. No hearing changes. Torsional nystagmus Dx—Hallpike maneuver	Epley maneuver by ENT or neurology (series of head movements to allow for repositioning of dislodged otoliths)
Ménière' s disease	Dilation of membranous labyrinth due to excess endolymph Classic symptoms = aural fullness, hearing loss, tinnitus & episodic vertigo lasting several hours	Medical—low sodium diet, antihistamines, benzodiazepenes thiazide, anticholinergics, intratympanic gentamicin. Surgery—endolymphatic sac decompression. Vestibular neurecomy, or labyrinthectomy
Vestibular neuritis	Proceded by viral respiratory illness. Severe vertigo lasting days to weeks. No hearing changes unless a complete viral labyrinthitis	Meclizine or benzodiazepines for severe symptoms

TABLE 13	*Continued*	
DISEASE	**CHARACTERISTICS**	**TREATMENT**
Acoustic neuroma (Figure 20)	CN VIII schwannoma commonly affects vestibular portion but can also affect cochlea Si/Sx = sudden deafness or hearing loss, tinnitus, rarely vertigo Dx = MRI with Gadolinium of cerebellopontine angle revealing enhancing lesion and possible surgical confirmation	Close observation by ENT. Surgical excision or local radiation
Migraines vertebrobasilar insufficiency (VBI), CVA, multiple sclerosis and neoplasm	Predisposing risk factors, usually no hearing changes. Can be acute or chronically progressive. VBI symptoms associated with elderly tilting head back, or shaving beard. Dx—Head CT/ MRI	Neurology consult. Disease specific treatment. Neoplasm and CVA must be ruled out if suspected

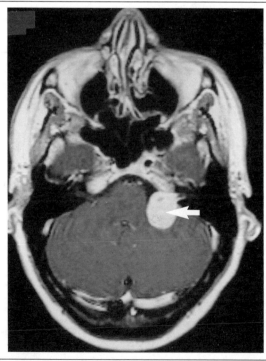

FIGURE 20 An MR Scan After Gadolinium Contrast Showing an Acoustic Neuroma

XVI. NOSE/SINUSES

A. Olfaction

1. 1° receptor → olfactory bulb → primary olfactory cortex → amygdala → entorhinal cortex → hippocampus

2. Bilateral anosmia can be due to trauma, viral disease

3. Unilateral anosmia is an early sign for a local tumor

B. Epistaxis

1. Most commonly involve nasal septum. Blood supply of septum; anterior and posterior ethmoidal arteries, sphenopalatine artery, nasal septal branch of labial artery, greater palatine artery. All converge in anterior septum in Little's area or Kiesselbach's plexus

2. 90% of bleeds occur at Kiesselbach's plexus (anterior nasal septum)

3. Note: Posterior bleeding more common in elderly

4. Blood supply to septum: anterior & posterior ethmoids → internal carotid artery, sphenopalatine, labial, and greater palatine → external carotid

5. **No. 1 cause of epistaxis in children is trauma (induced by exploring digits)**

6. Also precipitated by rhinitis, nasal mucosa dryness, septal deviation & bone spurs, alcohol, antiplatelet medication, and bleeding diathesis, cocaine abuse, and chronic hypertension, and hereditary hemorrhagic telangiectasia

7. Tx

   a. Direct pressure, topical nasal vasoconstrictors, i.e., oxymetazoline, phenylephrine, silver nitrate cautery (don't cauterize same location on both sides of septum to prevent septal perforation)

   b. Consider anterior nasal packing if unable to stop

   c. Five percent originate in posterior nasal cavity requiring packing to occlude choana. Patients with posterior packing or balloon should be admitted to hospital for airway observation. These patients are at increased risk for hypoventilation and decreased oxygen saturations

   d. Interventional radiology embolization of affected vessels

e. Surgical ligation of internal maxillary artery, ethmoidal arteries, or affected vessels to stop bleeding

f. Note: Patient's need to be placed on antistaphylococcal prophylaxis meds while nose is packed. Topical vasoconstrictors may be contraindicated in patients with hypertension

C. Sinusitis (see Figure 21)

1. Maxillary sinuses most commonly involved

2. Causes nasogastric tube, allergic rhinitis, rhinitis 2° to pregnancy, rhinitis medicamentosa (overuse of decongestants) & cocaine, nasal polyps obstructing drainage, and tumors

3. Potential complications of sinusitis include meningitis, abscess formation, orbital infection, and osteomyelitis

4. **Acute (<4 wk)**

   a. Most common organisms are *S. pneumoniae, H. influenzae,* and *Moraxella catarrhalis*

   b. Sx = purulent rhinorrhea, headache, pain on sinus palpation, pressure, fever, halitosis, anosmia, periorbital edema, tooth pain

   c. Tx = bactrim vs. augmented penicillins, decongestants, nasal saline irrigations

5. **Chronic (>3 month)**

   a. Most common organisms are *Bacteroides, Streptococcus spp., S. aureus,* and *Pseudomonas*

   b. Sx = same as for acute but last longer, also look for otitis media in children

   c. Tx = surgical correction of any sinus drainage obstructions, nasal steroids, antibiotics for acute exacerbations

   d. Complications of sinusitis

      1) Frontal sinuses—most dangerous complications occur here (see Figure 22 and Color Plate 8)

         a) Pott's puffy tumor—anterior extension of pus forming a subperiosteal abscess on forehead anterior to frontal sinus

         b) Orbital cellulitis/abscess from downward extension of pus

         c) Epidural/subdural/brain abscess from posterior extension of pus

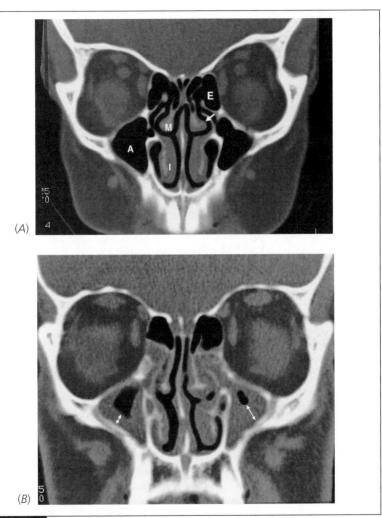

FIGURE 21   **Coronal CT Scan**

(A) Normal sinuses. Note the excellent demonstration of the bony margins. The arrow points to the middle meatus into which the maxillary antrum, frontal, anterior, and middle ethmoid sinuses drain. A = maxillary antrum; E = ethmoid sinus; I = inferior turbinate; M = middle turbinate. (B) Sinusitis. Mucosal thickening prevents drainage of the sinuses. Both antra are almost opaque. The arrows indicate mucosal thickening in the antra.

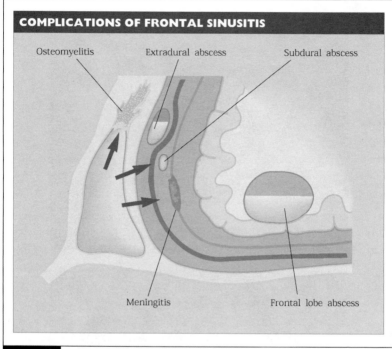

COMPLICATIONS OF FRONTAL SINUSITIS

Osteomyelitis   Extradural abscess   Subdural abscess

Meningitis   Frontal lobe abscess

FIGURE 22 **Complications of Frontal Sinusitis**

    d) Sagittal sinus thrombosis

  2) Spenoid sinuses

    a) Orbital apex syndrome—pressure on cranial nerves II, III, IV, and VI. Causing ophthalmoplegia and decreased vision

    b) Cavernous sinus thrombosis

6. Fungal

  a. Most common organisms are *Aspergillus spp.*, **& in diabetics think mucormycosis!**

  b. Usually seen in the immunocompromised (i.e., bone marrow transplant)

  c. Black nasal turbinates

  d. Vascular invasion noted in invasive fungal sinusitis, a deadly disease

  e. Tx = surgery and amphotericin

TABLE 14	Sinusitis		
	ORGANISMS	**Si/Sx**	**Tx**
Acute bacterial (<4 wk)	*S. pneumoniae, H. influenzae, Moraxella catarrhalis*	**Purulent rhinorrhea,** headache, **pain on sinus palpation,** fever, **halitosis,** anosmia, **tooth pain**	Bactrim, amoxicillin, decongestants
Chronic bacterial (>3 month)	*Bacteroides, Staph. aureus, Pseudomonas, Streptococcus spp.*	Same as for acute but lasts longer, also otitis media in children	Surgical correction of obstruction, nasal steroids
Fungal	*Aspergillus—* **diabetics get** mucormycosis!	Usually seen in the immunocompromised	Surgery & amphotericin

D. Nasal Tumors

1. **Juvenile angiofibroma**

   a. Benign vascular tumor causing unilateral epistaxis, usually seen in teenage boys

   b. Tx = radiotherapy or embolization & excision

2. **Polyps**

   a. Nasal & sinus polyps are commonly caused by allergy, asthma & chronic infection

   b. Polyps can obstruct airway & also encourage chronic sinus infections

   c. Tx = steroid nasal sprays and/or surgical excision

3. **Rhinophyma**

   a. Sebaceus hyperplasia of nasal dorsum

   b. Si/Sx = erythematous, large swollen nodular nose

   c. Commonly associated with Rosacea and cyclosporine use. No known cause; some theorize dermatoficum follicures

   d. Tx = CO_2 laser excision

4. **Wegener's granulomatosis**

a. Most common granulomatous systemic disease to affect nose

b. Pathology = necrotizing vasculitis with granuloma formation. Commonly c-ANCA positive (cytoplasmic anti-neutrophil cytoplasmic autoantibodies).

c. Si/Sx

1) Necrotizing granulomas of respiratory tract, glomerulitis, vasculitis

2) Nasal Sx = recurrent sinusitis, epistaxis, nasal obstruction

3) Other: gingival hyperplasia symptoms—subglottic stenosis, hemoptysis, proteinuria, and hematuria

4) Tx = azathioprine (Imuran), cyclophosphamide, or steroids

XVII. OUTPATIENT GASTROINTESTINAL COMPLAINTS

A. Dyspepsia

1. Si/Sx = upper abdominal pain, early satiety, postprandial abdominal bloating or distention, nausea, vomiting, often exacerbated by eating

2. DDx = peptic ulcer, gastroesophageal reflux disease (GERD), cancer, gastroparesis, malabsorption, intestinal parasite, drugs (e.g., NSAIDs), etc.

3. Dx = clinical

4. Tx = empiric for 4 wk, if Sx not relieved → endoscopy

5. Avoid caffeine, alcohol, cigarettes, NSAIDs, eat frequent small meals, stress reduction, maintain ideal body weight, elevate head of bed

6. H_2 blockers & antacids, or proton pump inhibitor

7. **Antibiotics for _H. pylori_ are NOT indicated for nonulcer dyspepsia**

B. Gastroesophageal Reflux Disease (GERD)

1. Causes = obesity, relaxed lower esophageal sphincter, esophageal dysmotility, hiatal hernia

2. Si/Sx = heartburn occurring 30–60 min postprandial & upon reclining, usually relieved by antacid self-administration, dyspepsia, postprandial burning sensation in esophagus, also regurgitation of gastric contents into the mouth

3. Atypical Si/Sx sometimes seen = asthma, chronic cough/laryngitis, atypical chest pain

4. Upper endoscopy → tissue damage but may be normal in 50% of cases

5. Dx = clinical, can confirm with ambulatory pH monitoring

6. Tx

   a. First line = lifestyle modifications: avoid lying down postprandial, avoid spicy foods & foods that delay gastric emptying, reduction of meal size, weight loss

   b. Second line = H_2-receptor antagonists—aim to discontinue in 8–12 wk

   c. Promotility agents may be comparable to H_2-antagonists

   d. Third line = proton pump inhibitors, reserve for refractory dz, often will require maintenance Tx since Sx return upon discontinuation

   e. Fourth line = surgical fundoplication, relieves Sx in 90% of pts, may be more cost-effective in younger pts or those with severe dz

7. Sequelae

   a. Barrett's esophagus—Chronic GERD → metaplasia from squamous to columnar epithelia in lower esophagus

      1) Requires close surveillance with endoscopy & aggressive Tx as 10% progress to adenocarcinoma

   b. Peptic stricture

      1) Results in gradual solid food dysphagia often with concurrent improvement of heartburn symptoms

      2) Endoscopy establishes diagnosis

      3) Tx = requires aggressive proton pump inhibitor & surgical opening if unresponsive

C. Hiatal Hernia

1. The majority of patients with reflux have hiatal hernia (80%)

2. Si/Sx = same as GERD

3. Dx = barium swallow to identify anatomic variations

4. There are two types of hiatal hernias

   a. Type I

      1) Sliding hiatal hernia is more common than the type II hernia

      2) It is the movement of the gastroesophageal junction & stomach up into the mediastinum

      3) Tx = medical as per GERD (see above) according to the degree of Sx present

   b. Type II

      1) Herniation of the stomach fundus through the diaphragm parallel to the esophagus

      2) Tx = mandatory surgical repair due to ↑ risk of strangulation

D. Achalasia

1. The most common motility disorder, affects 70% of pts with scleroderma

2. Loss of esophageal motility & failure of lower esophageal sphincter (LES) relaxation, may be caused by ganglionic degeneration or Chagas' disease, result in the dilatation of the proximal esophagus

3. Si/Sx = dysphagia of both solids & liquids, weight loss & repulsion of undigested foodstuffs that may produce a foul odor

4. May ↑ risk of esophageal CA because stasis promotes development of Barrett's esophagus

5. Dx

   a. Barium swallow → dilatation of the proximal esophagus with subsequent narrowing of the distal esophagus, studies may also reveal esophageal diverticula

   b. Manometry → ↑ LES pressure & diffuse esophageal spasm

6. Tx

    a. Endoscopic dilation of LES with balloon cures 80% of pts

    b. Alternative is a myotomy with a modified fundoplication

    c. Surgical Tx may be used for palliation in patients with scleroderma, who may experience dysphagia or severe reflux

E. Esophageal Diverticula (Zenker's Diverticulum) (see Figures 23 and 24)

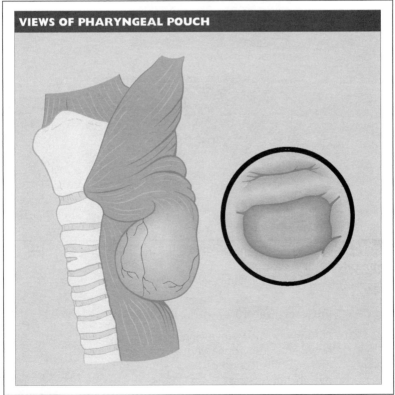

VIEWS OF PHARYNGEAL POUCH

FIGURE 23   **External and Endoscopic Views of the Pharyngeal Pouch**

Note how the pouch posteriorly compresses the opening of the esophagus.

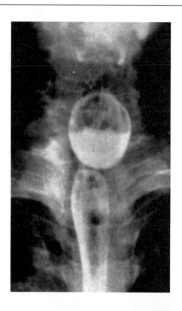

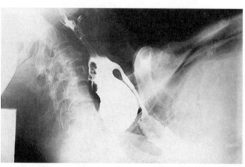

FIGURE 24   A Barium Swallow X-Ray Showing a Pharyngeal Pouch (top); Lateral View (bottom)

1. Proximal diverticula are usually Zenker's

2. Pulsion diverticula involving only the mucosa, located between the thyropharyngeal & cricopharyngeus muscle fibers (condition associated with muscle dysfunction/spasms)

3. Si/Sx = dysphagia, regurgitation of solid foods, choking, left-sided neck mass & halitosis

4. Dx = clinically + barium swallow

5. Tx = myotomy of cricopharyngeus muscle & removal of diverticulum

F. Esophageal Tumors

1. Squamous cell carcinoma

   a. Most common esophageal cancer, alcohol & tobacco synergistically ↑ risk of development

   b. Most commonly seen in men in the sixth decade of life

2. Adenocarcinoma

   a. Seen in pts with chronic reflux → Barrett's esophagus = squamous to columnar metaplasia

   b. 10% of Barrett's patients will develop adenocarcinoma

3. Si/Sx for both = **dysphagia**, weight loss, hoarseness, tracheoesophageal fistula, recurrent aspiration & may include symptoms of metastatic disease

4. Dx = barium study demonstrates **classic apple-core lesion**, Dx confirmed with endoscopy with biopsy to confirm diagnosis, CT of abdomen & chest is also performed to determine extent of spread

5. Tx = esophagectomy with gastric pull-up or colonic interposition with or without chemotherapy/radiation

6. Px poor unless resected prior to spread (very rare); however, palliation should be attempted to restore effective swallowing

G. Scleroderma (Progressive Systemic Sclerosis = PSS)

1. Systemic fibrosis affecting virtually every organ, female:male = 4:1

2. Can be diffuse disease (PSS) or more benign CREST syndrome

3. **CREST syndrome**

   a. **C**alcinosis = subcutaneous calcifications, often in fingers

   b. **R**aynaud's phenomenon, often the initial symptom

      1) Raynaud's = vasospasm of end-arterioles, frequently affecting digits

    2) Digits change colors from **white** → **blue** → **red**

        a) White = pallor due to vasospasm

        b) Blue = cyanosis due to prolonged vasospasm

        c) Red = reactive hyperemia when vasospasm ends

    3) Cold initiates (e.g., waking up in morning) & heat resolves (pts use hair dryers on hands & feet)

  c. **E**sophagitis

    1) Dysfunctional lower esophageal sphincter causes chronic reflux

    2) Esophageal strictures develop, Barrett's metaplasia occurs in one-third of patients

  d. **S**clerodactyly = fibrosed skin causes immobile digits & rigid facies (in severe cases affects limbs as well)

  e. **T**elangiectasias occur in mouth, on digits, face & trunk

4. Systemic Sx = tendinitis, severe flexion contractures, biliary cirrhosis, lung fibrosis causing dyspnea, myocardial fibrosis, renal artery fibrosis causing malignant hypertension

5. Lab = ⊕ANA in 95%, anti-Scl-70 has ↓ sensitivity but ↑ specificity, anticentromere is 80% sensitive for CREST syndrome

6. Tx = immunosuppressives for palliation, none are curative

H. Polymyositis

1. An autoinflammatory disorder of muscles & sometimes skin (dermatomyositis)

2. Female:male = 2:1, bimodal occurrence, in young children & geriatric populations

3. Sx = symmetric weakness/atrophy of proximal limb muscles, muscle aches, dysphonia (laryngeal muscle weakness), **dysphagia (esophageal dysfunction)**

4. Dermatomyositis presents with red-to-purple rash over face & neck called a "heliotropic rash"

5. Dx = proximal muscle weakness, ANA⊕ ↑serum creatine kinase, muscle biopsy → inflammatory changes

6. Main DDx = scleroderma

7. Tx = steroids (using CK to follow effectiveness), but can also use methotrexate or Cytoxan for resistant disease

XVIII. FACIAL NERVE DISORDERS

A. Facial Nerve (CN 7) Supplies Muscle of Facial Expression

1. It has five branches
   a. Temporal—**The***
   b. Zygomatic—**Zebra**
   c. Buccal—**Bought**
   d. Mandibular—**Me**
   e. Cervical—**Cerveza**

2. Lesions of upper motor neuron—patients demonstrate weakness of ipsilateral lower half of face and spare bilateral forehead
   a. Forehead receives bilateral supranuclear (corticalbulbar) innervation and therefore forehead not completely affected by unilateral upper motor neuron lesions

3. Lesions of lower motor neuron—patients demonstrate weakness of both upper and lower ipsilateral face

4. Patients with hyperacusis have lost stapedius reflex, which is innervated by CN VII

5. Special sensory (taste) to anterior two-thirds of tongue supplied by chorda tympani branch of CN VII

B. Unilateral Facial Palsy (Figure 25 and Color Plate 9)

1. Many potential causes. Careful follow up and evaluation needed

2. Trauma, neoplasm, infection, congenital, connective tissue disorders, and idiopathic (Bell's palsy)

C. Bell's Palsy

1. Idiopathic acute facial nerve paralysis is the most common cause of unilateral facial paralysis and is a diagnosis of exclusion

*Note: Compliments of Dr. Rudolpho Quintero

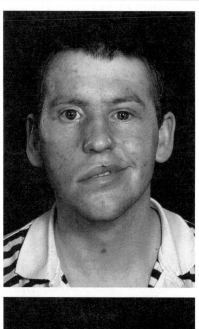

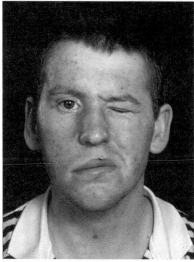

FIGURE 25 **Post-traumatic Right Facial Palsy**

Shown at rest and on attempted eye closure.

2. It is thought to be virally mediated and is usually self-limiting (putative cause is herpes simplex virus)

3. 80–90% of patients can expect good recovery within a few months. Complete paralysis of nerve at onset has a poorer prognosis. Tx = steroid, acyclovir

4. Can cause exposure keratitis—inflammation 2° to dry eyes caused by inability to close eyelids—natural tears

5. MRI with Gadolinium shows enhancement of cranial nerve VII perigeniculate region

D. Bilateral Facial Paralysis

1. An unusual disorder with a limited differential diagnosis

2. DDx = Lyme disease, sarcoidosis, temporal bone fractures, or Möbius syndrome (congenital facial paralysis & cranial nerve agenesis), Guillain-Barré, basilar meningitis, Wegener's, myasthenia gravis, HIV, and diabetes

3. Tx = diagnosis specific. Neuroimaging may be needed to evaluate facial nerve. ENT consult

E. Myasthenia Gravis (MG)

1. Caused by autoantibodies that block the postsynaptic acetylcholine receptor

2. The antibody blockade inhibits propagation of the action potential to the postsynaptic skeletal muscle

3. Most common in women in 20–30s or men in 50–60s

4. **Myasthenia often associated with thymomas & thyroid diseases, as well as other autoimmune diseases (e.g., lupus)**

5. Sx = **muscle weakness worse with use** (frequently patients complain of weakness at the end of the day)

   a. Classically affects facial muscles, causing diplopia or ptosis, altered smile, dysphagia

   b. Also causes proximal limb weakness

   c. Eventually can cause respiratory failure

6. Course can exacerbate or remit

   a. Often acutely exacerbated by infections

   b. Severe exacerbation called "crisis," can be fatal

7. Dx

    a. Tensilon screening test = trial of edrophonium (short-acting anticholinesterase inhibitor) → immediate ↑ in strength

    b. More definitive test is electromyelography with repetitive nerve stimulation, causing a >15% reduction in evoked action potential responses in stimulated muscle

8. DDx

    a. **Lambert-Eaton syndrome**

        1) Disorder seen in patients with small cell lung CA

        2) Caused by autoAbs to **pre**synaptic calcium channels

        3) Mimics myasthenia symptomatically

        4) Differs from MG in that Lambert-Eaton causes ↓ reflexes, autonomic dysfunction (xerostomia, impotence) & **Sx improve with muscle use (action potential strength increases upon repeated muscle stimulation)**

    b. Aminoglycoside use can exacerbate Sx in MG patients, or induce mild myasthenia Sx in normal people

    c. Penicillamine can induce mild myasthenia, but it is reversible with cessation of drug use

9. Tx = anticholinesterase inhibitors (e.g., pyridostigmine) first line

    a. Steroids, cyclophosphamide, azathioprine for ↑ severe dz

    b. Plasmapheresis temporarily alleviates Sx by removing the blocking antibody

    c. Resection of thymoma can be curative in patients with both the neoplasm & myasthenia

    d. In addition, even in pts with no thymus neoplasm, resection of a normal thymus causes symptomatic improvement in 85% of patients, & may be curative in up to 35%

F. Sarcoidosis

1. Diffuse, systemic disorder of unknown etiology, which may be infectious or autoimmune in nature

2. **African Americans are three times more likely to develop than Caucasians**, peaks in 20–40s

3. Fifty percent pts present with incidental finding on CXR in an aSx person

4. Other presentations include fevers, chills, night sweats, weight loss, cough, dyspnea, rash, arthralgia, and blurry vision (uveitis)

5. 90% of patients develop abnormal CXR at some point

6. **Classic CXR finding is bilateral hilar adenopathy, sarcoidosis should be suspected in ANY patient with this finding on CXR**

7. Can affect ANY organ system

   a. CNS → CN palsy, classically CN VII (can be bilateral facial nerve palsy)

   b. **Eye → uveitis (can be bilateral), this classic Sx mandates immediate Ophtho consult & aggressive Tx (see below)**

   c. Cardiac → heart blocks, arrhythmias, constrictive pericarditis

   d. Lung → typically a restrictive defect

   e. GI → ↑ AST/ALT, CT → granulomas in liver, cholestasis

   f. Renal → nephrolithiasis (granulomas secrete 1-α-hydroxylase, causing ↑ production of 1,25-OH-vit D → hypercalcemia)

   g. Endocrine → classic cause of diabetes insipidus due to pituitary involvement, ↑ vitamin D as above

   h. Hematologic → bone marrow involvement & splenic sequestration causes anemia, thrombocytopenia, leukopenia

   i. Derm → various rashes, including erythema nodosum

8. Dx is clinical; however, finding of **noncaseating granulomas on Bx (often of lymph nodes) is HIGHLY suggestive if no other explanation is found for the granulomas** (e.g., fungal infections)

9. Lab: 50% pts have ↑ angiotensin converting enzyme level—used to follow Tx (will ↓ with Tx) but not Dx due to ↓ sensitivity

10. Tx = prednisone (first line), but 50% pts spontaneously remit, so only Tx if 1) eye/heart involved, 2) dz does not remit after months

11. Treatment

a. ENT follow-up

b. To prevent corneal ulceration—artificial tears, gold weight in eyelid, or surgical closure of the eyelids

c. Steroids and acyclovir have occasionally been found to be helpful in Bell's palsy

d. Surgical decompression or nerve grafting may be needed

G. Cranial Nerves III–XII Located in the Brain Stem

1. Motor nuclei lie close to midline, sensory nuclei tend to lie more laterally

2. CN III lesion = downward/outward eye deviation & ptosis (levator palpebrae superioris)

   a. Associated Edinger-Westphal nucleus damage causes loss of parasympathetic innervation of pupillary constrictor & ciliary muscles, leads to pupillary dilation, loss of accommodation

   b. **Fixed, dilated pupil is classic presentation**

3. CN IV lesion = **contralateral eye deviates up & in (CN IV is the only nerve that crosses the midline)**

4. CN V nucleus is gigantic, understand the corneal reflex & masticator reflex

   a. CN V sensory afferents → main sensory nuclei V → CN VII → orbicular oculi muscles

   b. Type Ia masticator muscle spindle afferents via V_3 → CN V motor nuclei → masseter muscle

   c. Lesions of V sensory lead to ipsilateral loss of pain & temperature sensation of face

5. CN VI lesion = medial deviation of eye, may also see CN VII involvement due to proximity of VII nerve to body of VI

6. CN VII lesions of **two varieties**: nuclear lesions or corticobulbar lesions

   a. CN VII lesions → also known as Bell's palsies, paralysis of facial muscles, loss of anterior 2/3 taste, loss of lacrimation & salivation, & can also involve CN VI

   b. Corticobulbar fibers innervate **all cranial motor nuclei bilaterally, except CN VII**

      1) CN VII fibers to upper facial muscles do receive bilateral corticobulbar innervation

2) CN VII fibers to lower facial muscles **only receive contralateral cortical innervation**

3) Consequence: **a unilateral lesion of cortex can lead to contralateral lower facial muscle paralysis, while no deficit will be noticed in the upper facial muscles**

7. CN VIII lesions: path is so complex may see no deficit due to redundant innervation

8. CN IX lesions = unilateral loss of swallowing, taste & gag reflex

9. CN X lesions = unilateral loss of palatal elevation, taste & laryngeal dysfunction

10. CN XI lesions = unilateral loss of trapezius, sternocleidomastoid function

11. CN XII lesion = deviation of tongue to **same side as lesion**

H. Cranial Nerves in Skull Passageways

1. Superior orbital fissure → CN 3, 4, 5_1, 6

2. Foramen rotundum → CN 5_2

3. Foramen ovale → CN 5_3

4. Internal auditory meatus → CN 7, 8

5. Jugular foramen → CN 9, 10, 11

6. Cavernous sinus → CN 3, 4, 5_1, 6 (all that control extraocular motion)

XIX. ORAL CAVITY DISORDERS (See Figures 26 and 27 and Color Plates 10 and 11)

A. Cancer

1. Tongue

   a. Squamous cell carcinoma most common

   b. Sx = nonhealing ulcer on tongue, swollen tongue

   c. Tx = surgical excision and/or radiation

2. Lip

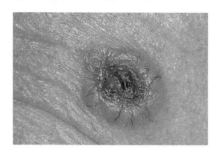

FIGURE 26   Classic Crateriform Basal Cell Carcinoma. Ulcerating Nodule

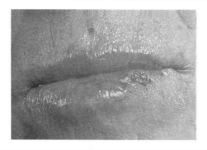

FIGURE 27   Squamous Cell Carcinoma of the Lip (Early Ulcer)

  a. Squamous cell carcinoma most common, and usually affecting lower lip

  b. Basal cell more commonly affects upper lip

  c. Si/Sx = easily visible nonhealing lesions. Basal cell has characteristic rodent ulcer appearance with telangiectasias

  d. Tx = surgical excision and/or radiation

B. Blistering Disorders

  1. Pemphigus vulgaris (PG)

     a. PG is a rare autoimmune disorder, **affecting 20–40 yr olds**

     b. **IgG autoantibodies are directed against an epidermal cement substance** (desmoglein III, a cadherin)

     c. IgG titers correlate with course of disease

    d. Destruction of cement substance leads to intraepidermal acantholysis **with sparing of basal layer**

    e. Demonstrated by classic **immunofluorescence surrounding epidermal cells showing "tombstone fluorescent pattern"**

    f. PE shows **flaccid epidermal bullae** that easily slough off leaving large denuded areas of skin (Nikolsky's sign), subject to 2° infxn

    g. **Can be fatal if not treated**

    h. Tx = steroids

2. Bullous pemphigoid (BP)

    a. Resembles PG but much less severe clinically

    b. Common autoimmune disease affecting **mostly the elderly**

    c. **IgG antibodies directed against an antigen in the epidermal basement membrane**

    d. Demonstrated by **immunofluorescence as a linear band along the basement membrane** (lamina lucida layer)

    e. Increased eosinophils can usually be seen in dermis

    f. PE shows **hard, tense bullae** that do not rupture easily & usually heal without scarring if uninfected

3. Erythema multiforme

    a. Characterized by **target-like lesions**

    b. Caused by a hypersensitivity response to certain drugs or infections, or to systemic disorders such as malignancy or collagen vascular disease

    c. Commonly lesions accompany a herpes eruption (prevent eruption of herpes with acyclovir & prevent E. multiforme)

    d. Lesions come in many forms, hence the name "multiforme"

    e. **A severe febrile form (sometimes fatal) is Stevens-Johnson syndrome, where hemorrhagic crusting also affects lips & oral mucosa**

4. Cutaneous Porphyria Tarda

    a. Autosomal dominant defect in heme synthesis (50% ↓ in uroporphyrinogen decarboxylase activity in RBC & liver)

    b. Si/Sx = blisters on sun-exposed areas of face & hands, ↑ facial hair around temples & cheeks, under Woods lamp **urine fluoresces with distinctive orange-pink color due to ↑ levels of uroporphyrins**

    c. **No abdominal pain** (differentiates from other porphyrias)

    d. Course = remitting/relapsing, exacerbations due to hepatitis virus, hepatoma, alcohol abuse, estrogen, sunlight

    e. Tx = sunscreen, phlebotomy, chloroquine, no EtOH

5. Herpes labialis (cold sores) usually due to herpes simplex (HSV-1)

    a. Usually related to recent stressor (infection, fever, life)

    b. Si/Sx = itching, pain, blisters, ulceration, self-limiting

    c. Tx = usually self-limiting, antivirals can be used to shorten course if started early

    d. DDx = aphthous stomatitis (canker sore) caused by *S. sanguis*, iron, B$_{12}$, or folate deficiency, and idiopathic

        1) Most common type of oral lesion usually apppearing on mobile tissue of oral cavity

        2) Si/Sx = similar to HSV, nonblistering, painful

        3) Tx = self-limiting, topical steroids, tetracycline for 7 days may be used for *S. sanguis*

6. Behçet's syndrome

    a. Multisystem inflammatory disorder that chronically recurs

    b. Classically presents with painful oral & genital, eye and skin ulcers

    c. Also can see arthritis, vasculitis, & severe neurologic lesions

    d. Classic dermatologic Sx = oral lesions and **circinate balanitis** (serpiginous, moist plaques on glans of penis) & **keratoderma blennorrhagicum** (crusting papules with central erosion, **look like mollusk shell**)

    e. HLA-BW51, B5, B27, B12 commonly affected

    f. Bx = mononuclear infiltration

    g. Tx = prednisone during flare-ups

C. Systemic Disorders

1. Crohn's disease (inflammatory bowel disease)

   a. A GI inflammatory disease that may be infectious in nature

   b. Affects any part of GI from mouth to rectum, but usually the intestines

   c. Si/Sx = abdominal pain, diarrhea, malabsorption, fever, stricture causing obstruction, fistulae, see below for extraintestinal manifestations

   d. Dx = colonoscopy with biopsy of affected areas → transmural, **noncaseating granulomas, cobblestone mucosal morphology, skip lesions, creeping fat on gross dissection is pathognomonic**

   e. Tx

      1) Sulfasalazine (5-ASA), better for colonic dz but also helps in small bowel

      2) Steroids for acute exacerbation, but no effect on underlying dz

      3) Immunotherapy (azathioprine & mercaptopurine)—useful in pts with unresponsive dz

      4) Newest Tx are tumor necrosis factor (TNF) antagonists, etanercept (recombinant TNF factor), and infliximab (anti-TNF monoclonal antibody)

2. Familial polyposis syndromes

   a. Familial adenomatous polyposis (FAP)

      1) Si/Sx = autosomal dominant inheritance of APC gene, abundant polyps throughout the colon & rectum beginning at puberty

      2) **Gardner's syndrome** consists of polyposis, desmoid tumors, **osteomas of mandible or skull, & sebaceous cysts**

      3) Turcot's syndrome is polyposis with medulloblastoma or glioma

      4) Dx = family Hx, colonoscopy, presence of congenital hypertrophy of retinal pigment epithelium predicts FAP with 97% sensitivity

       5) Tx = colectomy & upper GI endoscopy to rule out gastroduodenal lesions—a favored operation is an abdominal colectomy, mucosal proctectomy, & ileoanal anastomosis

  b. **Peutz-Jeghers syndrome**

      1) Si/Sx = autosomal dominant inheritance, nonneoplastic hamartomatous polyps in stomach, small intestine & colon, skin & mucous membrane hyperpigmentation, **particularly freckles on lips, risk of developing CA in other tissues** (e.g., breast, pancreas)

      2) Dx = clinical & family Hx

      3) Tx = careful, regular monitoring for malignancy

3. Systemic Lupus Erythematosus

  a. Systemic autoimmune disorder, female:male = 9:1

  b. Si/Sx include fever, polyarthritis, skin lesions, hemolytic anemia, thrombocytopenia, splenomegaly, pleural effusions, pericarditis (serositis), Libman-Sacks endocarditis, nephrosis or nephritis, thrombosis & a variety of neurologic disorders

  c. Labs

      1) **Antinuclear antibody (ANA) sensitive (>98%) but not specific**

      2) **Anti-double-stranded-DNA (anti-ds-DNA) antibodies are 99% specific but less sensitive**

      3) Anti-Smith (anti-Sm) antibodies are highly specific but not sensitive

      4) Anti-Ro antibodies are ⊕ in 50% of ANA-negative lupus, so they are good fail-safe if clinical suspicion of lupus is high, but ANA is negative

      5) Antiribosomal P & antineuronal antibodies correlate with risk for cerebral involvement of lupus (lupus cerebritis)

      6) Antiphospholipid autoantibodies cause false positive lab tests in SLE

         a) **SLE patients frequently have false ⊕ RPR/VDRL tests for syphilis** due to anticardiolipin antibodies

         b) **SLE patients frequently have elevated PTT coagulation times (lupus anticoagulant antibody)**

        i) PTT is falsely ↑ because the lupus anticoagulant antibody binds to phospholipid, which initiates clotting in the test tube

        ii) **Despite the PTT test & the name *lupus anticoagulant antibody*, SLE patients are THROMBOGENIC, because antiphospholipid antibodies cause coagulation *in vivo***

d. **Mnemonic for SLE diagnosis:** DOPAMINE RASH

    1) **D**iscoid lupus = characteristic circular, erythematous macules with scales, postinflammatory central depigmentation

    2) **O**ral aphthous ulcers (can be nasopharyngeal as well)

    3) **P**hotosensitivity

    4) **A**rthritis (typically hands, wrists, knees)

    5) **M**alar rash = classic butterfly macule on cheeks

    6) **I**mmunologic criteria = anti-ds-DNA, anti-Sm Ab, anti-Ro Ab, anti-La Ab (⊕ ANA is a separate criteria)

    7) **N**eurologic changes = psychosis, personality change, seizures

    8) **E**SR rate is almost always elevated (**Note:** this is not 1 of the 11 diagnostic criteria, but it is a frequent lab finding)

    9) **R**enal disease → nephritic or nephrotic syndrome

    10) **A**NA ⊕

    11) **S**erositis (pleurisy, pericarditis)

    12) **H**ematologic dz = hemolytic anemia, thrombocytopenia, leukopenia

e. Drug-induced SLE

    1) Drugs = procainamide, hydralazine, sulfonamides, INH, cephalosporin

    2) **Lab → antihistone antibodies**, differentiating from idiopathic SLE

    3) Resolves upon cessation of offending drug

f. Tx = NSAIDs, prednisone, cyclophosphamide depending on severity of dz

    1) Px = variable & difficult to predict over long term, but 10-yr survival is excellent, **renal dz is a poor Px indicator**

D. Oral Candidiasis (Thrush)

1. Occurs in diabetics, immunocompromised, young children, and patients on antibiotics and steroids

2. Si/Sx = white-curd-like lesions on an erythamatous base in oral cavity and oropharynx, odynophagia, and burning tongue pain

3. Tx = nystatin swish and swallow, mycelex troches, and "magic mouthwash"

   a. Magic mouthwash—30 mL of Mylanta (Maalox), 30 mL of benadryl elixir, 30 mL of 2% viscous lidocaine. Swish and spit with 5 mL of this solution every 4–6 hr as needed

   b. Other combinations used to include carafate, and nystatin

E. Acute Necrotizing Gingivitis = "Trench Mouth" or "Vincent's Infection"

1. Caused by fusiform bacilli & spirochetes

2. Si/Sx = malaise, +/– fever, painful/bleeding gingiva, fetid breath

3. Dx = **punched out lesion, gray membrane, bleed easily to touch is pathognomonic**

4. Tx = débridement, analgesic, salt water rinse, penicillin if acute

F. Ludwig's Angina

1. Infectious cellulitis usually spreading from infected tooth

2. Submaxillary, sublingual spaces affected causing a swelling of anterior floor of mouth

3. Si/Sx = fever, pain, drooling, edema, erythema of upper neck under the chin, can cause airway compromise due to swelling of tongue. May extend from neck into superior mediastinum

4. Tx = airway, airway, airway, immediate tracheotomy may be safest way to go. IV antibiotics, airway protection, surgical debridement and drainage of fluid collections and multiple incisions of mylohyoid muscle to prevent reacumulation

5. Note: Extension into superior mediastinum can occur via carotid sheath migration

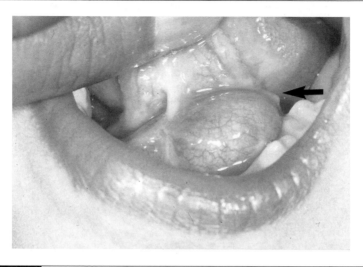

FIGURE 28   Sublingual Retention Cyst

G. Ranula (Latin for Frog) (see Figure 28)

1. Floor of mouth sialocele (retention cyst) presenting as a painless swelling under tongue appears like a small toad under tongue

2. Secondary to sublingual gland salivary duct obstruction

3. Tx = may resolve spontaneously or need surgical excision of duct and sublingual gland

H. Fetor Oris

1. Foul-smelling breath

2. Common in dental/tonsillar infections (peritonsillar abscess) & lung or sinus infections

I. Trismus (Lockjaw)

1. Caused by spasm of muscles of mastication, so person has difficulty opening mouth

2. Seen in tetanus & in other dzs that cause local or widespread muscle spasms: rabies, scleroderma, or tonsillar infection

3. Tx = disease specific

J. Temporomandibular Joint (TMJ) Disorder

1. A disorder of temporomandibular joint can be congenital or acquired

2. Si/Sx = TMJ clicking or popping when opening mouth wide, otalgia, mandible pain at rest, locking of jaw in open or closed position, trismus, joint tenderness on palpation, malocclusion, and night-time teeth grinding

3. Patients commonly present complaining of an ear pain that has never been properly treated. Symptoms worsening after a recent visit to dentist

4. Dx = CT or MRI of TMJ, clinical physical exam

5. Tx = soft diet, rest, stress reduction, NSAIDs, muscle relaxants, splints, oral surgery consult

6. Jaw locked and dislocated. Treat by pushing downward and posteriorly on mandible

K. Angioedema (Angioneurotic Edema)

1. Swelling of tongue, lips, and oral cavity

2. Can be acutely mediated by IgE, or commonly caused by angiotensin converting enzyme (ACE) inhibitors use

3. Also seen in a functional or quantitative C1 esterase inhibitor deficiency (hereditary angioedema)

4. Tx = treat for allergic reaction with diphenhydramine and steroids. Patients with C1 esterase inhibitor deficiency. May use Danazol, which increases C1 esterase, or aminocaproic acid, which decreases complement activation

5. **Differential diagnosis**

   a. **Melkersson-Rosenthal syndrome**

      1) Persistent nonremitting agioedema like swelling of lips and perioral tissues

      2) Bx reveals a granulomatous process

      3) Tx = steroids clofazamine

   b. **Hypersensitivity reactions**

      1) **Allergic Hypersensitivity (Type 1)**

         a) IgE-mediated, due to release of vasoactive mediators from mast cells & basophils

         b) Examples = allergies, anaphylaxis, atopic diseases

2) **Cytotoxic Hypersensitivity (Type 2)**

a) Antibody-mediated, typically IgG binds to antigen on target cell surface, inducing complement lysis, ADCC, or phagocytosis

b) Examples = autoimmune hemolytic anemia, erythroblastosis fetalis, pemphigus, Goodpasture's disease, penicillin-induced anemia, hyperacute transplant rejection

3) **Immune Complex Hypersensitivity (Type 3, Arthus Reaction)**

a) Antigen-antibody complexes bind complement, which attracts neutrophils & induces lytic enzyme release, causing tissue damage

b) Examples = serum sickness, SLE systemic findings, postinfectious glomerulonephritis

4) **Delayed Type Hypersensitivity (DTH, Type 4)**

a) TH1-directed, macrophage-mediated, no antibodies involved

b) Examples = contact dermatitis, acute/chronic transplant rejection, TB & poison ivy

L. Tumors

1. Papilloma = most common tumor of oral mucosa, occurs in mouth

2. Fibroma results from chronic irritation

3. Epulis = benign tumor of gingivae, usually is reparative growth

4. Leukoplakia = irregular white patches caused by hyperkeratosis 2° to chronic irritation

   a. Usually benign, may be precancerous dysplasia

   b. **Note, oral hairy leukoplakia (OHL)** is seen virtually exclusively in HIV+ patients

   c. OHL = raised, white, patch with tiny hair-like spikes, caused by EBV or possibly other herpes

   d. OHL = cannot scrape off with tongue blade, no response to antifungals, biopsy is EBV+

    5. Ameloblastoma

        a. Enamel precursor tumor, appears before age 35

        b. **Oral cancer is squamous cell CA, involves tongue in 50% cases, risks = smoking, alcohol,** chewing betel nuts

XX. SALIVARY GLAND DISORDERS

A. Anatomy

    1. Major salivary glands (see Figure 29)

        a. Parotid

           1) Drained by Stensen's duct

           2) Serous secretory cells

           3) Most common site of salivary gland tumors (80–90%)

           4) Most common benign tumor—pleomorphic adenoma

           5) Most common malignant tumor—mucoepidermoid carcinoma

              a) Facial nerve involvement more commonly associated with malignant disease

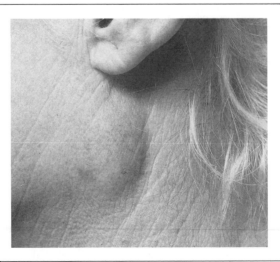

FIGURE 29   A Pleomorphic Adenoma in the Tail of the Parotid Gland

   b. Submandibular

     1) Drained by Wharton's duct

     2) Both serous and mucous secretory cells

     3) Second most common site of salivary gland tumors

     4) Tumors are benign 50%, malignant 50%

   c. Sublingual

     1) Drains into floor of mouth

     2) Mostly mucus-secreting cells

     3) Tumors are benign 40%, malignant 60%

   d. Thousands of minor salivary glands throughout oral cavity and pharynx

     1) Tumors of minor salivary glands are more commonly malignant

     2) In children hemangiomas are the most common salivary gland neoplasms

B. Disorders

1. Sialadenitis

   a. Inflammation of salivary glands due to infection, inflammation, or sialolithiasis (obstructive stone)

   b. Dx = CT scan with contrast, sialography if obstruction suspected or if stones are radioluscent on CT

   c. Tx = antistaphyloccocal antibiotics, massage, warm compresses, pain meds, hydaration, sialogogues—items that promote saliva production such as lemons, or dry lemon juice powder

   d. ENT referral if Sx unresolved or worsening

2. Parotitis

   a. Bilateral parotid swelling—usually caused by a viral infection, mumps, HIV, Sjogren's, or bulimia

   b. Unilateral swelling most commonly caused by *Staphylococcus aureus*. Patients usually presents with facial swelling, pain, and erythema. Massaging of parotid gland allows pus to drain from Stensen's duct

   c. If Sx persists or facial nerve involved consider tumor

    d. CT scan with contrast to rule out abscess or to evaluate for enlarged lymph nodes or stone

    e. IV hydration, antibiotics, and sialagogues such as lemon wedges to encourage gland function. Massage and hot compresses to affected gland

    f. Fine needle aspirate (FNA) of gland to evaluate for tumor. If nondiagnostic, superficial parotidectomy needed

3. Sjogren's syndrome (SS)

    a. An autoinflammatory disorder associated with **HLA-DR3**

    b. Classic triad of Sjogren's

        1) **Keratoconjunctivitis sicca** = dry eyes

        2) **Xerostomia** = lack of salivary secretions, often due to parotitis

        3) **Inflammatory arthritis**, usually less severe than pure RA

        4) Concomitant presence of two of the triad is diagnostic

    c. Some variants affect only the eyes or mouth (1° SS)

    d. Associated systemic Sx = pancreatitis, fibrinous pericarditis, CN V sensory neuropathy, renal tubular acidosis, 40-fold ↑ in lymphoma incidence

    e. Lab → ANA ⊕, anti-Ro/anti-La Ab ⊕ ("SSA/SSB Abs"), 70% are RF ⊕, 70% have ↑ ESR, anemia/leukopenia

    f. Tx = steroids, cyclophosphamide for refractory disease

4. Mumps

    a. Paramyxovirus, spread by saliva droplet, more communicable than measles or chickenpox

    b. Gland swelling lasts 5–9 days, incidence peaks in winter & early spring, usually in 5–15 yr/o

    c. Sx/Si = chill, anorexia, malaise, headache, low-mod fever 12–24 hr prior to parotitis

    d. During parotitis, fever elevates, painful chewing & swallowing

    e. Px = excellent, Tx = symptomatic

        1) Rare sequelae = orchitis, meningoencephalitis, Bell's palsy, pancreatitis

    f. DDx = suppurative (strep/diphtheria/typhus), Mikulicz's syndrome, tumor, stone, Sjogren's syndrome

1) Mikulicz's syndrome = chronic, painless, parotid/lacrimal swelling, unknown etiology but occurs during TB, sarcoid, SLE, leukemia & lymphosarcoma

2) Sjogren's syndrome causes xerostomia & parotid swelling

5. Mucocele

a. Cystic pool of mucus lined by granulation tissue, not epithelium, near salivary gland

b. Results from leakage of damaged mucous ducts

XXI. NECK/THROAT DISORDERS

A. Pharyngitis/Tonsillitis (Sore Throat)

1. Waldeyer's ring—oropharyngeal lymphoid tissue composed of adenoids, lateral pharyngeal bands, palatine tonsil, lingual tonsils. Common sites of inflammation

2. Bacterial

a. *Streptococcus pyogenes* (group A Strep) & *Staph*. Most common organisms

1) Presents with severe pain in throat, temperatures of 103°F or more, mucosa is bright red, edematous, white or yellow exudate can be seen on tonsils

2) Tx = penicillin

b. Membranous (diphtheria) caused by *Corynebacterium diphtheriae*

1) **Pathognomonic physical finding = a patch of gray membrane on the tonsils extending down into the throat**

2) Potential consequences include airway occlusion by membrane & myocarditis

3) **Tx is antitoxin as quickly as possible to prevent cardiac damage!** Antibiotics (erythromycin) are given to reduce bacterial load

3. Fungal

a. Oral thrush or moniliasis, caused by *Candida spp.*

     1) Presents with white, cheesy patches on pharynx, tongue, & buccal mucosa

     2) Common in AIDS patients

     3) Tx = nystatin liquid, swish around mouth & swallow

4. Viral

  a. Adenovirus

     1) Infects mucosa of respiratory tract, gastrointestinal tract, & conjunctiva

     2) Causes pharyngoconjunctival fever, a self-limiting dz

  b. Epstein-Barr virus (EBV)

     1) Infectious mononucleosis is difficult to distinguish from strep throat

     2) More systemic findings are typically seen in mono

     3) Si/Sx = generalized lymphadenopathy, exudative tonsillitis, palatal petechiae & splenomegaly, **atypical lymphocytes** seen on blood smear

     4) Lab testing shows ⊕ **heterophile antibody** in contrast to mono caused by CMV, which is heterophile antibody negative

     5) **Skin rash** commonly occurs in patients mistakenly treated with antibiotics (penicillin, ampicillin)

  c. Parainfluenza virus

     1) The major cause of laryngotracheobronchitis (croup)

     2) Seen mostly in children under 5 yr

     3) **Presents with barking cough worse at night**, pharyngitis, inspiratory stridor

     4) Classic x-ray finding is a steeple sign on anterior x-ray of neck

  d. Coxsackie A virus

     1) Causes herpangina—classic presentation is sudden fever, pharyngitis & body ache

     2) Two days after onset, tender vesicles erupt along tonsillar pillars, uvula, & soft palate

     3) Vesicles ulcerate after several days

     4) Occurs in epidemics in infants & children

     5) Self-limiting disease, Tx = symptomatic

B. Peritonsillar Abscess (Quinsy)

1. Loculation of pus in the peritonsilar space (between tonsil and superior constrictor)

2. May be related to previous tonsillar infection, dental caries, or allergies

3. May be caused by anaerobic bacteria, but mostly caused by same agents seen in pharyngitis & tonsillitis

4. Si/Sx = fever, drooling, odynophagia, trismus & a muffled voice. Soft palate & uvula are displaced and peritonsillar fluctuant swelling that is extremely painful to touch

5. Tx = airway stabilization, incision & drainage, antibiotic treatment and fluids. Quinsy tonsillectomy immediately vs. wait 6 wk and perform tonsillectomy

C. Lemierre's syndrome

1. Thrombophleitis of internal jugular (IJ) vein

2. Usually secondary to oropharyngeal infection with anaerobic gram negative rods. Most commonly *Fusobacterium necrophorum*

3. Si/ Sx = severe odynophagia, dysphagia, fevers, chills, rigors, neck swelling or pain. Occasionaly a palpable cord may be felt along IJ clot. Septic emboli commonly metastasize to lungs forming cavitations and abscesses

4. Tx = longterm IV antibiotics with clindamycin, and possible surgical drainage of abscesses or surgical ligation of clot if unresponsive to antibioitics and continued emboli

D. Retropharyngeal Abscess (see Figure 30)

1. An abscess formed from breakdown and necrosis of enlarged lympnodes in retropharyngeal space

2. More common in children and usually following a severe pharyngeal infection or longstanding upper respiratory infection c lymphadenitis

3. Si/Sx = toxic appearing, drooling stridor, high fever, head tilted to one side, dysphagia, odynophagia. Unilateral bulging noted within oropharynx

4. Dx = CT scan with contrast, lateral neck, airway flouroscopy

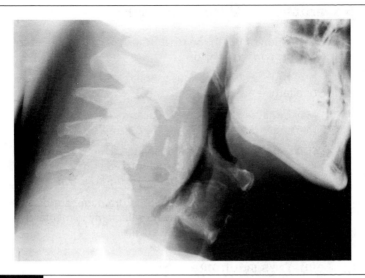

FIGURE 30 Retropharyngeal Abscess in an Adult Secondary to a
Foreign Body

5. Tx = Stabilize airway, IV antibiotics, ENT consult and surgery
   if Sx don't improve or patient unstable

E. Epiglottitis (Supraglottitis)

1. Presents in children, caused by *H. influenzae* type B.
   Examine airway in operating room to prevent
   bronchospasm and airway obstruction

2. Rare now due to efficacy of HiB vaccine

3. Presents with acute airway obstruction, sudden airway
   emergency, inspiratory stridor, drooling, high fever,
   dysphagia, no cough, neck pain

4. Rarely seen in adults, usually caused by *S. pneumoniae*
   or S. aureus

5. Classic x-ray finding is **"thumb sign"** on lateral neck film

6. Tx = immediate airway intubation, stabilize airway and
   observe, IV antibiotics

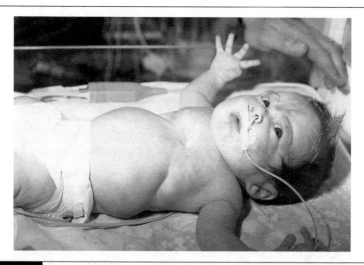

FIGURE 31   Baby with Severe Upper Airway Obstruction

Note the sternal recession and paradoxical abdominal movement.

F. Stridor (see Figure 31)

1. Laudible high-pitched noisey breathing caused by air turbulence

2. Inspiratory stridor—supraglottis affected

3. Biphasic stridor (inspiratory/expiratory)—glottic or subglottic narrowing

4. Most common pediatric noninfectious cause—laryngomalacia (see Figure 32)

5. Most common pediatric infectious cause is viral croup

6. Other causes—subglottic hemangioma, polyps, foreign body, vascular rings. Vocal cord paralysis (see Figure 33)

7. Tx = stabilize airway. Humidified oxygen, steroids, and nebulized racemic epinephrine as needed

8. ENT consult, x-ray, lateral neck and chest x-ray, and airway fluoroscopy, to evaluate airway if stable

9. Immediate stabilization of airway if unstable. Direct laryngoscopy and bronchoscopy to further evaluate airway once patient stabilized

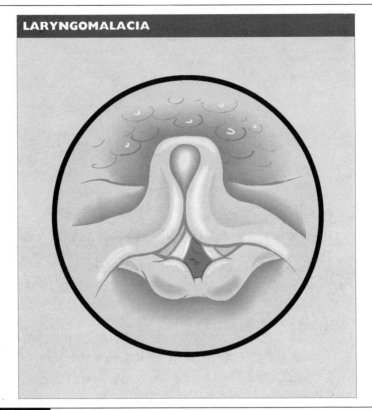

LARYNGOMALACIA

FIGURE 32 **Laryngomalacia**

Note the insuction of the supraglottic structures, causing airway narrowing.

G. Sleep Apnea—periods of apnea occuring during sleep

1. Most commonly obstructive-increased inspiratory effort that fails to result in increased airflow

2. Patients are usually obese, heavy snorers who awake after a gasp for air. Pts complain of excessive daytime sleepiness. Spouse complains of loud snoring

3. Can lead to pulmonary hypertension, and sudden death

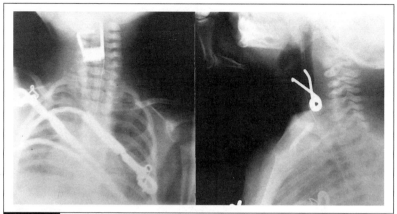

FIGURE 33 **An Unexpected Foreign Body in a 6-Week-Old Baby, Causing Stridor**

The x-ray illustrates the need for lateral x-ray films of the neck in any child with stridor, since the foreign body was not visible on a chest x-ray.

4. Tx = weight loss, continuous positive airway pressure (CPAP) at night to maintain patent airway. Surgery if no relief and severely affecting lifestyle or danger to life

5. Rule out central apnea where no respiratory effort exist, and obtain sleep study to evaluate for extent and occurrence of oxygen desaturation episodes

H. Cervical Lymphadenitis

1. Enlarged lymph nodes in neck

2. Bilateral lymphadenopathy is usually viral

3. Unilateral lymphadenopathy is usually bacterial

4. Common organisms include *S. aureus* & group A & B Strep (*pyogenes* & *agalactiae*)

5. Differentiate from cat scratch fever, often caused by *Bartonella henselae*, which is inoculated into patient after scratch by young cats

6. Hodgkin's lymphoma can also present unilaterally

7. Scrofula = localized lymphadenopathy related to tuberculosis infection

8. *Actinomyces israelii* → localized cervical nodes that have bright red sinuses & drain pus containing "sulfur-like granules"

9. Kawasaki's syndrome also causes cervical lymphadenopathy

I. Adenoiditis (see Figure 34)

1. Commonly seen in young children

2. Si/Sx = frequent otitis media episodes, snoring at night, constant mouth breathers, constant nasal congeation, and hypernasal voice

3. Patients develop an adenoid facies from always having mouth open

4. Tx = surgical removal of adenoids

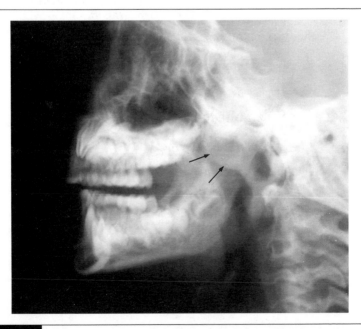

FIGURE 34 A Lateral Soft Tissue X-Ray Showing Adenoid Enlargement

TABLE 15	Pharyngitis		
DISEASE	**Si/Sx**	**Dx**	**Tx**
Group A Strep throat	High fever, **severe throat pain without cough**, edematous **tonsils with white or yellow exudate, cervical adenopathy**	• H&P 50% accurate • Antigen agglutination kit for screening • Throat swab culture is gold standard	Penicillin to prevent acute rheumatic fever
Membranous (diphtheria)	High fever, dysphagia, drooling, **can cause respiratory failure** (airway occlusion)	• **Pathognomonic gray membrane on tonsils extending into throat**	**STAT antitoxin**
Fungal (*Candida*)	Dysphagia, sore throat with white, cheesy patches in oropharynx (oral thrush), **seen in AIDS & small children**	• Clinical or endoscopy	Nystatin liquid, swish & swallow
Adenovirus	**Pharyngoconjunctival fever (fever, red eye, sore throat)**	• Clinical	Supportive
Mononucleosis (EBV)	Generalized lymphadenopathy, exudative tonsillitis, palatal petechiae & splenomegaly	• ⊕ **Heterophile antibody** • **Skin rash** occurs in pts given ampicillin	Supportive
Herpangina (coxsackie A)	Fever, pharyngitis, body ache, tender vesicles along tonsils, uvula & soft palate	• Clinical	Supportive

J. Kawasaki's Syndrome

1. Vasculitis that affects medium-sized vessels

2. Coronary artery aneurysms are deadly components of this dz

3. Most commonly presents in children 6 months → 4 years, usually in Asians

4. Patients present with high, unresponsive fever for at least 5 days

TABLE 16	Neck Mass Differential Diagnosis		
DISEASE	**CHARACTERISTICS**	**Dx FINDINGS**	**Tx**
	Congenital		
Torticollis	• Lateral deviation of head due to hypertrophy of unilateral sternocleidomastoid • Can be congenital, neoplasm, infection, trauma, degenerative disease, or drug toxicity (particularly D_2 blockers = phenothiazines) pseudotumor of infancy	Rock hard knot in the sternocleido-mastoid that is easily confused with the hyoid palpation	Muscle relaxants &/or surgical repair
Thyroglossal duct cyst	• **Midline** congenital cysts, which usually present in childhood	**Cysts elevate upon swallowing**	Surgical removal
Branchial cleft cyst	• **Lateral** congenital cysts, which usually do not present until adulthood, when they become infected or inflamed cholesterol crystals	**Do not elevate upon swallowing** Aspirate contains	Surgical excision
Cystic hygroma	• Lymphatic malformation that usually presents within first 2 years of life • **Lateral or midline**	Translucent, benign mass painless, soft & compressible	Surgical excision
Dermoid cyst	• **Lateral or midline** • Soft, fluctuant mass composed of an overgrowth of epithelium	**No elevation with swallowing**	Surgical excision
Carotid body tumor = paraganglioma	• Palpable mass at bifurcation of common carotid artery • Not a vascular tumor, but originate from neural crest cells in the carotid body within the carotid sheath • Rule of 10: 10% malignant, 10% familial, 10% secrete catecholamines	**Pressure on tumor can cause bradycardia & dizziniess**	Surgical excision

		Dx	
DISEASE	**CHARACTERISTICS**	**FINDINGS**	**Tx**
TABLE 16 *Continued*			

		Dx	
Acquired-Inflammatory			
Cervical lymphadenitis	• Bilateral lymphadenopathy is usually viral, caused by EBV, CMV, or HIV • Unilateral is usually bacterial, caused by *S. aureus*, group A & B Strep, other causes • Cat scratch fever (*Bartonella henselae*), transmitted via scratch of young cats • Scrofula due to miliary tuberculosis • *Actinomyces israelii* → sinuses drain pus containing "sulfur granules" • Kawasaki's syndrome • Hodgkin's lymphoma	Fine-needle aspirate & culture	Per cause: Viral → supportive, bacteria →IV antibiotics, Kawasaki's → aspirin, Lymphoma → chemotherapy

5. Additional Si/Sx: **CRASH** mneumonic

 a. **C**onjunctivitis

 b. **R**ash, primarily truncal, which can resemble any type of rash previously discussed

 c. **A**neurysms of coronary arteries

 d. **S**trawberry tongue, crusting of lips, fissuring of mouth, & oropharyngeal erythema

 e. **H**ands & feet show induration, erythema of palms & soles, desquamation of fingers & toes

 f. Associated Sx = arthritis, diarrhea, hydrops of gallbladder, single node adenopathy (>1.5 cm in neck)

 g. Labs show ↑ ESR, C-reactive protein, **thrombocytosis** (600,000–1,800,000)

6. Tx = ↑ dose aspirin, **steroids contraindicated in these pts**

7. Intravenous immunoglobulin may prevent cardiac disease

K. Malignant Neoplasms of Head & Neck

1. Most commonly squamous cell carcinoma

2. Careful and thorough head and neck physical exam

3. Panendoscopy indicated for evaluation of most head and neck cancers

   a. Bronchoscopy

   b. Laryngoscopy

   c. Esophagoscopy

   d. Chest x-ray/CT of chest

L. Malignant Melanoma

1. Increasing in age-adjusted incidence

2. Most common in lightly pigmented individuals, sun exposure is an important pathogenic factor

3. Can arise from melanoma cells or dysplastic nevus cells

4. Growth can occur in all directions, but usually begins by growing radially or laterally within the epidermis & superficial dermis (papillary zone), from where it does not metastasize

5. **Melanomas kill people because of high rate of metastasis**

6. Clinically, lesion removal during lateral growth phase imparts a better prognosis due to far lower rate of metastasis

7. Vertical growth phase consists of extension into the deep dermis

   a. **Lesions during this phase have a markedly increased capacity to metastasize**

   b. Most important Px factor = depth of lesion within dermis

8. Four types: superficial spreading, acral (nails), lentiginous (Hutchinson freckle), & nodular

9. Nodular melanoma begins with vertical phase, has the worst Px

10. Physical exam focuses on the **ABCDE**s

    a. **A**symmetry: benign lesions are usually symmetrical, melanomas are usually asymmetrical

b. **B**order: benign lesions have smooth borders, melanomas have irregular borders

c. **C**olor: benign lesions have only one color, melanomas have more than one color

d. **D**iameter: benign lesions are usually <6 mm in diameter, melanoma usually >6 mm in diameter

e. **E**levation: melanoma is usually elevated & palpable, especially when malignant

11. Tx = excision & perhaps regional lymph node dissection, consider adjunctive chemotherapy for systemic treatment or prophylaxis (generally not very effective)

M. Basal Cell Carcinoma

1. **Most common malignant skin tumor**

2. Typically seen in sun-exposed areas

3. **Rodent ulcer usually seen on face, with pearly borders & fine telangiectasias**

4. Not usually found on lips

5. Histologically look for palisade arrangement of nuclei & tumor islands

6. Tx = excision, **these lesions virtually never metastasize**

N. Squamous Cell Carcinoma

1. Mostly occurring on sun-exposed areas

2. **Actinic keratosis (AK) frequently precedes this form of skin cancer**

a. AK = rough keratin plaques, usually seen on sun-exposed areas

b. Lips, scalp, cheeks, & ear are commonly affected

3. Squamous CA more likely to metastasize than basal cell CA, but not as likely as melanoma

4. **Histologically look for keratin pearls**

5. Tx = AK removal (using cryotherapy) before it converts to squamous cell CA, & excision of squamous cell CA before metastasis

O. Neurocutaneous Syndromes (Phakomatoses)

1. Tuberous sclerosis

   a. Autosomal dominant skin & CNS syndrome

   b. Skin findings include hypomelanotic macules (hypopig-mented, described as ash leaf patches), leathery cuta-neous thickening (Shagreen spots), & adenoma sebaceum of the face

2. Neurofibromatosis (NF)

   a. Autosomal dominant

   b. Presents with café-au-lait spots, neurofibromas, meningiomas, acoustic schwannomas, kyphoscoliosis

   c. NF 2 presents with bilateral acoustic neuromas (CN VIII)

3. Sturge–Weber

   a. No genetic pattern

   b. Presents with port-wine hemangioma of face, in the distribution of the trigeminal nerve, which also involves the meninges

   c. Mental retardation & seizures accompany this disorder

4. Von Hippel-Lindau syndrome

   a. Autosomal dominant syndrome of diffuse hemangiomas

   b. ↑ risk of developing renal cell CA, also associated with increased secretion of erythropoietin causing polycythemia

P. Kaposi's Sarcoma

1. Endothelial cell cancer caused by human herpes virus 8

2. Appears as red/purple plaques or nodules on skin & mucosa

3. Frequently also affects GI viscera & lungs

4. Almost exclusively seen in homosexual AIDS patients (not in AIDS patients who contracted HIV by IV drug abuse)

5. Other HIV-related ENT disorders include oral candida, bilateral facial palsy, trigeminal neuralgia, and erythema multiforme

6. No effective Tx, although may regress with strong HIV Tx

Q. Rhabdomyosarcoma

1. Most common in children in head, neck, & urogenital area

2. Can occur in conjunction with tuberous sclerosis

3. Tx = surgical excision, but often fails due to rapid spread of the tumor

R. Lymphoma

1. General characteristics

   a. Lymphomas are solid tumors of the lymphoid system (lymph node, tonsils, GI tract, spleen, & liver)

   b. Can commonly affect Waldeyer's ring and present with large nontender, firm, fixed lymph nodes in the neck

   c. These are differentiated from reactive lymph nodes, which are tender, soft, moveable, & smaller

   d. Typically lymphoma is not found in bone marrow like leukemia

   e. Two major types of lymphoma are Hodgkin's & non-Hodgkin's

2. Non-Hodgkin's lymphoma (NHL)

   a. Description

      1) Histology → diffuse or follicular (nodular)

      2) Grade → low, intermediate, or high, related to degree of differentiation of cell type

      3) Morphology → large or small cell with multiple variants (e.g., cleaved or noncleaved)

   b. Follicular vs. diffuse type

      1) Follicular (nodular) type

         a) Rare in children, better Px than diffuse counterpart

         b) Is a B-cell type

         c) Those with small cells do better than large cells

      2) Diffuse type

         a) More aggressive than nodular

         b) Either B-cell or T-cell type

         c) Highly aggressive (high grade) are always diffuse

c. Grade

1) Low grade → small lymphocytic, follicular small cleaved cell, follicular mixed small cleaved

2) Intermediate grade → follicular large cell, diffuse small cleaved cell, diffuse mixed/small/large cell types

3) High grade

   a) The most aggressive NHLs; all are histologically diffuse types

   b) Types

   i) Immunoblastic type seen in immunocompromised

   ii) Lymphoblastic involves mediastinum & bone marrow, is TdT positive & has T-cell markers

   iii) **Small noncleaved cell = Burkitt's lymphoma**

      a)) B-cell type, closely linked to Epstein–Barr virus

      b)) African Burkitt's (endemic) involves jaw bones

      c)) US form involves abdomen more commonly

      d)) **Classic histologic description is the "starry sky pattern,"** caused by dark background of densely packed lymphocytes (sky) with light colored spots in them caused by scattered macrophages (the stars)

      e)) Translocation of *c-myc* from chromosome 8 to chromosome 14 Ig heavy chain locus

d. Cutaneous T-cell lymphoma (CTCL, mycosis fungoides)

1) Slowly progressive CD4 T-cell lymphoma of the skin, usually occurring in elderly

2) **Classic histologic description → cells contain cerebriform nuclei** (nucleus looks like cerebral gyri)

3) Often presents with systemic erythroderma, a total body erythematous & pruritic rash, which can precede clinically apparent malignancy by years

4) Leukemic phase of this disease is called "Sézary syndrome"

e. Angiocentric T-cell lymphoma

      1) Two subtypes = nasal T-cell lymphoma (lethal midline granuloma) & pulmonary angiocentric lymphoma (Wegener's granulomatosis)

      2) Nasal T-cell lymphoma is EBV associated

      3) Both are highly lethal, nonresponsive to chemotherapy

      4) Classic presentation = large mass that when biopsied is nondiagnostic due to large areas of necrosis within mass

      5) Can cause airway compromise by local compression/edema

      6) Tx = palliative radiation therapy

3. Hodgkin's lymphoma

  a. Occurs in a bimodal age distribution, young men (women for nodular sclerosis type, see below) & geriatric population

  b. EBV infection is present in up to 50% of cases

  c. Si/Sx resemble inflammatory disorder, **classic Pel-Epstein fevers** (fevers wax & wane over weeks), chills, night sweats, weight loss, leukocytosis, **in some pts Sx worsen with alcohol intake**

  d. Reed–Sternberg (RS) cells

      1) Possibly the malignant cell of Hodgkin's

      2) **Classically appear as binucleated giant cells ("owl eyes") with eosinophilic inclusions**

      3) **One variation is Lacunar cell, a mononucleated giant cell**

      4) Dz severity is proportional to number of RS cells seen in tumor

  e. Rye classification contains four variants

      1) Lymphocytic predominance is least frequently occurring, a B-cell type

      2) Mixed cellularity

        a) Most frequently occurring type

        b) Histology → lymphocytes, eosinophils, RS cells, plasma cells

      3) Nodular sclerosis

      a) More frequent in women

      b) Histology

          i) **Nodular division of lymph nodes by fibrous bands**

          ii) **Lacunar cell RS variant**

    4) Lymphocyte depletion

      a) Poorest prognosis

      b) Histology → frequent necrosis, many RS cells

  f. Clinical staging more closely linked to Px than histologic type

    1) Stage I = one lymph node involved

    2) Stage II = two or more lymph nodes on same side of diaphragm

    3) Stage III = involvement on both sides of diaphragm

    4) Stage IV = disseminated, ≥1 organ or extranodal tissue involved

    5) Type A = systemic symptoms absent

    6) Type B = systemic symptoms present (e.g., fever, night sweats, unexpected weight loss >10%)

XXII. THYROID

A. Physiology

1. TRH secreted by hypothalamus, stimulates TSH secretion by anterior pituitary

2. The α-subunit of TSH is identical to that of FSH, LH, & HCG—the β-subunit gives specificity

3. Thyroid hormones = thyroxin (T4) & tri-iodothyronine (T3)

4. Synthesis depends upon sufficient quantities of iodine from diet

5. Iodine absorbed in upper GI tract, enters blood stream, is trapped by an active transport system in thyroid follicular cells

6. Iodine + thyroid peroxidase → iodide + hydrogen peroxide + tyrosine → MIT/DIT, MIT + DIT → T3, DIT + DIT → T4

7. TSH binds to thyroid cell membrane receptors, activates adenylate cyclase, ↑ cAMP, & ↑ thyroid hormone

8. Serum T3 & T4 are bound to thyroid-binding globulin (TBG)

9. In peripheral tissues T4 is converted to T3 or reverse T3 (rT3)

10. T3 is four times more biologically active than T4, rT3 is inactive

11. In the perinatal period maturation of CNS is absolutely dependent on thyroid hormone

    a. Deficiency causes irreversible mental retardation

    b. All neonates undergo mandatory screening for hypothyroidism

B. Congenital Thyroid Disease

1. Thyroid develops as outpouching of endoderm at base of tongue

2. Gland migrates caudally to its final resting position in the developed infant

3. During this migration, the gland remains connected to its starting point by the thyroglossal duct (site is marked in the developed organism by the foramen cecum)

4. Thyroglossal duct normally involutes during development, but cysts can present along tract of the duct during adolescence (or, rarely, adulthood) as thyroglossal cysts

5. Thyroglossal cysts are ALWAYS midline (main DDx—branchial cleft cysts, which lie laterally on the neck, & dermoid cysts)

6. **Thyroglossal cysts elevate with swallowing or sticking tongue out, whereas others do not**

7. Islets of ectopic thyroid tissue may lie anywhere along the tract of the resorbed thyroglossal duct

C. Goiter

1. Enlargement of the thyroid gland implies NOTHING about thyroid function

2. Potential causes = normal physiologic enlargement (puberty/pregnancy), dietary iodine deficiency, inflammation, gland hyperfunction, goitrogens (compounds in food or drugs that suppress gland's hormone production)

3. The term *toxic* implies hyperthyroidism (↑ levels of serum thyroxine)

D. Hyperthyroidism

1. General

   a. Causes = Grave's disease, iatrogenic, Plummer's disease, adenoma, subacute thyroiditis, apathetic hyperthyroidism, struma ovarii, silent thyroiditis, 2° disease

   b. Si/Sx of hyperthyroidism = tachycardia, **isolated systolic hypertension**, tremor, a-fib, anxiety, diaphoresis, weight loss with increased appetite, insomnia/**fatigue**, diarrhea, **exophthalmus, heat intolerance**

   c. T4/3 levels fluctuate with changes in TBG levels, so serum levels are not strictly useful to measure

      1) Pregnancy elevates TBG levels via estrogen, falsely elevating the lab value of the serum T4

      2) Nephrotic syndrome & cirrhosis lower TBG levels, falsely lowering T4 levels

2. Grave's disease (diffuse toxic goiter) is the most common cause (90% of US hyperthyroid cases)

   a. Grave's is seen in young adults & is eight times more common in females than males

   b. Caused by idiopathic autoimmune response to the TSH receptor, autoantibody stimulates the receptor

   c. **Grave's disease Si/Sx include two characteristic findings only seen in hyperthyroid due to Grave's: infiltrative ophthalmopathy & pretibial myxedema**

   d. **Infiltrative ophthalmopathy**

      1) Similar to exophthalmus, but blurry/double vision is acquired due to weakness of ocular muscles

      2) Whereas simple exophthalmus resolves when the thyrotoxicosis is cured, infiltrative ophthalmopathy may not be reversible (waxes & wanes, with no correlation to the pt's thyroid status)

      3) Because of the above finding, it is clear that thyrotoxicosis is not responsible for infiltrative ophthalmopathy—instead it is hypothesized that autoantibodies damage retrobulbar tissues

e. **Pretibial myxedema**

    1) Dermopathy, usually on the shins, characterized by brawny, pruritic, nonpitting edema

    2) Unlike infiltrative exophthalmus, pretibial myxedema often spontaneously remits after months to years

3. Plummer's disease (toxic multinodular goiter)

    a. Due to multiple foci of thyroid tissue that cease responding to T4 feedback inhibition

    b. More common in older people, as opposed to Grave's

    c. Dx

        1) Physical exam → feel multiple nodules whereas Grave's is diffusely enlarged

        2) Radioactive iodine uptake tests show hot nodules, with abnormally cold background gland due to suppression of normal tissue by overactive nodules

4. Thyroid adenoma due to overproduction of hormone by tumor in the gland

5. Subacute thyroiditis (granulomatous, giant cell, or de Quervain's thyroiditis)

    a. **BEWARE:** This disease presents with hyperthyroidism that later turns into hypothyroidism

    b. Due to inflammation of the thyroid gland with early spilling of hormone from the damaged gland

    c. See below under Hypothyroid, for more

6. Apathetic hyperthyroidism is idiopathic condition seen in elderly where only Sx is often intractable CHF with atrial fibrillation

7. Silent thyroiditis

    a. Occurs mostly in women, often in postpartum period

    b. Characterized by mild, transient thyrotoxicosis with goiter

8. Struma ovarii

    a. An ovarian teratoma containing ectopic thyroid tissue

    b. Usually benign, 5% pts develop clinical hyperthyroidism

9. 2° hyperthyroidism very rare, due to hypersecretion of TSH from pituitary (3° even rarer, due to ↑ TRH)

10. Labs

    a. TBG sites are low in hyperthyroidism & T3RU (T3 resin uptake) is high in hyperthyroidism

    b. Radioiodine uptake ↑ in Grave's, Plummer's, toxic adenoma

    c. Radioiodine uptake ↓ in subacute thyroiditis, exogenous hormone, struma ovarii

11. Treat hyperthyroidism medically or surgically

    a. Medicine = propylthiouracil or methimazole, both of which block thyroid production of hormone

    b. Drug therapy induces remission in 1 month to 2 yr (up to 50% of time), so life-long therapy is not necessary

    c. Radioiodine is first line for Grave's: radioactive iodine is concentrated in the gland & destroys it, resolving the diffuse hyperthyroid state

    d. If the above fail → surgical excision (of adenoma or entire gland)

12. Thyroid storm is the most extreme manifestation of hyperthyroidism

    a. Not a separate disease entity in & of itself

    b. Due to exacerbation of hyperthyroidism of above causes

    c. Precipitated by surgery, infection, & anesthesia

    d. Causes high fever, dehydration, cardiac arrhythmias, high output cardiac failure, coma, & 25% mortality rate

    e. Tx with high-dose β-blockers, supportive measures

E. Hypothyroid

1. Congenital hypothyroidism

    a. Due to 2° agenesis of thyroid or defect in enzymes

    b. **T4 is crucial during first 2 yr of life for normal brain development**

    c. Birth Hx → normal Apgars, prolonged jaundice (↑ indirect bilirubin)

    d. Si/Sx = presents at 6–12 wk old with poor feeding, lethargy, **hypotonia, coarse facial features, large protruding tongue**, hoarse cry, constipation, developmental delay

    e. Dx = ↓ T4, ↑ TSH

    f. Tx = levothyroxine replacement

    g. **If Dx delayed beyond 6 wk, child will be mentally retarded**

    h. Newborn screening is mandatory by law

2. General

    a. Causes include Hashimoto's, subacute thyroiditis, Riedel's thyroiditis, silent thyroiditis

    b. Si/Sx = **cold intolerance**, weight gain, **low energy,** husky voice, mental slowness, constipation, thick/coarse hair, puffiness of face/eyelids/hands (**myxedema**), prolonged relaxation phase of deep tendon reflexes

    c. Myxedema due to accumulation of hyaluronic acid (hydrophilic) glycosaminoglycan & water in every organ

3. Hashimoto's disease

    a. Autoimmune lymphocytic infiltration of the thyroid gland

    b. Ratio 8:1 in women to men, usually between ages of 30 and 50

    c. Other autoimmune diseases often accompany (SLE, RA, Sjogren's, etc.: **Schmidt's syndrome** = Hashimoto's + endocrine disorders such as diabetes or Addison's disease)

    d. Dx by hypothyroid Sx/Si & labs, also look for antimicrosomal antibodies (antithyroid peroxidase antibodies)

    e. Tx by life-long synthroid

    f. Fine-needle aspirate → lymphoid follicles with germinal centers & **Hurthle** cells (follicular epithelial cells with basophilic cytoplasmic inclusions)

    g. Minority of glands → fibrous with parenchymal obliteration

4. Subacute thyroiditis

    a. Seen following flu-like illness with sore throat & fevers

    b. Pain often exists in jaw/teeth, can be confused with dental disease, aggravated by swallowing or turning head

    c. Early inflammation leads to spillage of T4, looks like hyperthyroid, only late leads to hypothyroid

    d. Elevated ESR is characteristic

    e. Disease is most often self-limiting & resolves without consequences after weeks to months

    f. Usually does not progress to the stage of clinical hypothyroidism

    g. Tx with aspirin, only with cortisol in very severe disease

5. Riedel's thyroiditis

    a. A very rare idiopathic disorder where entire thyroid gland is replaced by fibrous tissue

    b. Can be confused with malignancy

6. Myxedema coma

    a. **The only emergency hypothyroid condition**

    b. Spontaneous or precipitated by cold exposure, infection, analgesia, sedative drug use, respiratory failure, or other severe illness

    c. Si/Sx = overt hypothyroidism, stupor, coma, convulsive seizures, hypotension, hypoventilation

7. Neonatal hypothyroidism = cretinism

    a. Presents with respiratory difficulties, cyanosis, persistent jaundice, poor feeding, hoarse crying, macroglossia, & mental retardation

    b. Tx = lifetime thyroxine

F. Malignancy

1. Terms *hot* & *cold* used to describe nodules, refer to whether or not the nodules take up iodine (i.e., are they functionally active or not)

2. Hot nodules are rarely cancerous, usually seen in elderly, soft to palpation, ultrasound (Utz) shows cystic mass, thyroid scan shows autonomously functioning nodule

3. Cold nodule

    a. Has a greater potential of being malignant

    b. More common in women

    c. Nodule is firm to palpation, often accompanied by vocal cord paralysis, Utz shows solid mass

4. Papillary CA

    a. **The most common cancer of thyroid**

    b. Good Px, 85% 5-yr survival, spread is indolent, via lymph nodes

    c. Pathologically distinguished by **ground glass Orphan Annie nucleus & psammoma bodies** (other psammoma body dz = serous papillary cystadenocarcinoma of ovary, mesothelioma, meningioma)

5. Medullary CA

    a. Has intermediate prognosis

    b. Cancer of parafollicular "C" cells that are derived from the ultimobranchial bodies (cells of branchial pouch 5)

    c. Secretes calcitonin, can Dx & follow dz with this blood assay

6. Follicular CA

    a. Good Px, commonly blood-borne metastases to bone & lungs

7. Anaplastic CA has one of the poorest Px of any cancer (0% survival at 5 yr)

    a. Note: Thyroid Nodule—fine needle aspirate, surgical excison

G. The Multiple Endocrine Neoplasia Syndromes

1. MEN Type I (Wermer's syndrome)

    a. Hyperplasia or tumors of parathyroid, adrenal cortex, pancreas & pituitary

    b. **The 3(4) P's:** **P**ituitary (**P**rolactinoma most common), **P**arathyroid, **P**ancreatoma (most often gastrinoma causing Zollinger-Ellison syndrome)

2. MEN Type IIa (Sipple's syndrome)

    a. Pheochromocytoma, medullary CA of the thyroid, hyperparathyroidism due to hyperplasia or tumor

    b. This is the only type with both thyroid CA & parathyroid tumor

    c. Associated with mutation of the *ret* oncogene

3. MEN Type IIb ("MEN Type III")

   a. Pheochromocytoma, medullary CA & multiple mucocutaneous neuromas, particularly of the GI tract

   b. Only type that does not include hyperparathyroidism

   c. Like MEN IIa, associated with mutation of *ret* oncogene (interesting note: Hirschsprung's disease is a congenital colonic atresia 2° to failure of myenteric plexus neuronal development & is associated with loss of function mutations in the *ret* oncogene

XXIII. ENT TRAUMA

A. General

1. Trauma is the major cause of death in those under age 40

2. Management broken into primary & secondary surveys

B. Primary Survey = ABCDE

1. **A** = **A**irway

   a. All pts immobilized due to ↑ risk of spinal injury

   b. Maintain airway with jaw thrust or mandible/tongue traction, protecting cervical spine

   c. If pt is likely to vomit, position them in a slightly lateral & head-down position to prevent aspiration

   d. If airway cannot be established, two large bore (14-gauge) needles can be inserted into the cricothyroid membrane

   e. Do not perform tracheotomy in the field or ambulance

   f. Unconscious patients need endotracheal (ET) tube!

2. **B** = **B**reathing

   a. Assess chest expansion, breath sounds, respiratory rate, rib fractures, sub-Q emphysema, & penetrating wounds

   b. Life-threatening injuries to the lungs or thoracic cavity are:

1) Tension pneumothorax → contralateral mediastinal shift, distended neck veins (↑ CVP), hypotension, ↓ breath sounds on one side & hyperresonance on the other side, Tx = immediate chest tube or 14-gauge needle puncture of affected side

2) Open pneumothorax → Tx = immediate closure of the wound with dressings & placement of a chest tube

3) Flail chest → caused by multiple rib fractures that form a free-floating segment of chest wall that moves paradoxically to the rest of the chest wall, resulting in an inability to generate sufficient inspiratory or expiratory pressure to drive ventilation, Tx = intubation with mechanical ventilation

4) Massive hemothorax → injury to the great vessels with subsequent hemorrhage into the thoracic cavity, Tx = chest tube, surgical control of the bleeding site

3. **C** = **C**irculation

a. Two large bore IVs placed in upper extremities (if possible)

b. For severe shock, place a central venous line

c. O-negative blood on stand-by for any suspected significant hemorrhage

4. **D** = **D**isability

a. Neurologic disability assessed by history, careful neurologic examination (Glasgow Coma Scale), laboratory tests (blood alcohol level, blood cultures, blood glucose, ammonia, electrolytes, & urinalysis) & skull x-rays

b. Loss of consciousness

1) DDx = **AEIOU TIPS** = **A**lcohol, **E**pilepsy, **E**nvironment (temp), **I**nsulin (+/–), **O**verdose, **U**remia (electrolytes), **T**rauma, **I**nfection, **P**sychogenic, **S**troke

2) Tx = coma cocktail = dextrose, thiamine, naloxone, & O_2

c. ↑ ICP → HTN, bradycardia, & bradypnea = Cushing's triad

d. Tx = ventilation to keep $PaCO_2$ at 30–40 mmHg, controlling fever, administration of osmotic diuretics (mannitol), corticosteroids & even bony decompression (burr hole)

5. **E** = **E**xposure

a. Remove all clothes without moving pt (cut off if necessary)

b. Examine all skin surfaces & back for possible exit wounds

c. Ensure patient not at risk for hypothermia (small children)

C. Secondary Survey

1. Identify all injuries, examine all body orifices

2. Periorbital & mastoid hematomas ("raccoon eyes" & Battle's sign), hemotympanum & CSF otorrhea/rhinorrhea → basilar skull fractures

3. The Glasgow Coma Scale should be performed

4. Deaths from abdominal trauma are usually from sepsis due to hollow viscous perforation or hemorrhage if major vessels are penetrated

5. Diagnostic peritoneal lavage, abdominal Utz, or CT scan (if pt stable) suggests abdominal injury, if pt unstable Dx is by surgical laparotomy, Tx = surgical hemostasis

6. If blood noted at urethra, perform retrograde urethrogram before placement of a bladder catheter, hematuria suggests significant retroperitoneal injury & requires CT scan for evaluation, take pt to OR for surgical exploration if unstable

7. Check for compartment syndrome of extremities, Si/Sx = tense, pale, paralyzed, paresthetic & painful extremity, Tx = fasciotomy

D. Shock

1. Table 17

2. Table 18

3. Shock in trauma can be neurogenic or hypovolemic

TABLE 17	Differential Diagnosis of Shock		
TYPE	**CARDIAC OUTPUT**	**PULMONARY CAPILLARY WEDGE PRESSURE**	**PERIPHERAL VASCULAR RESISTANCE**
Hypovolemic	↓	↓	↑
Cardiogenic	↓	↑	↑
Septic	↑	↓	↓

TABLE 18	Correction of Defect in Shock	
TYPE	**DEFECT**	**FIRST-LINE TREATMENT**
Hypovolemic	↓ preload	2 large bore IVs, crystalloid or colloid infusions (see Fluids and Electrolytes above), replace blood losses with the **3 for 1** rule = give 3 L of fluid per liter of blood loss
Cardiogenic	Myocardial failure	Pressors—dobutamine first line, can add dopamine and/or norepinephrine, supplemental O_2
Septic	↓ peripheral vascular resistance	Norepinephrine to vasoconstrict peripheral arterioles, prevent progression to multiple organ dysfunction syndrome (MODS), give IV antibiotics as indicated, supplemental O_2

TABLE 19	Body Surface Area in Burns			
Palm of hand	1%	Upper extremities*	9%
Head & neck*	9%	Lower extremities*	18%
Anterior trunk*	18%	Genital area*	1%
Posterior trunk*	18%		

*In adults.

4. Neurogenic due to blood pooling in splanchnic bed & muscle from loss of autonomic innervation

5. Tx = usually self-limiting, can be managed by placing pt in supine or Trendelenburg position

E. Burns (Table 19)

1. Partial thickness

   a. 1° & 2° burns are limited to epidermis & superficial dermis

   b. Si/Sx = skin is red, blistered, edematous, skin underneath blister is pink or white in appearance, very painful

   c. Infection may convert to full-thickness burns

2. Full thickness

    a. 3° & 4° burns affect all layers of skin & subcutaneous tissues

    b. Si/Sx = skin is initially painless, dry, white, charred, cracked, insensate

    c. 4° burns also involve muscle & bone

    d. All full-thickness burns require surgical treatment

    e. % of body surface area (BSA) affected

    f. Tx = resuscitation, monitor fluid status, remove eschars

        1) Consider any facial burns or burning of nasal hairs as a potential candidate for ARDS & airway compromise

        2) Fluid resuscitation

            a) Parkland formula = % BSA $\times$ weight (kg) $\times$ 4, formula used to calculate volume of crystalloid needed

            b) Give half of fluid in first 8 hr, remainder given over the next 16 hr

        3) CXR to r/o inhalation injury

    g. Labs → PT/PTT, CBC, type & cross, ABGs, electrolytes, UA

        1) Irrigate & débride wound, IV & topical antibiotics (silver sulfadiazine, mafenide, polysporin), tetanus prophylaxis & stress ulcer prophylaxis

        2) Transfer to burn center if pt is very young or old, burns >20% BSA, full-thickness burns >5% BSA, coexisting chemical or electrical injury, facial burns, or pre-existing medical problems

        3) Make pt NPO until bowel function returns, pt will have extremely ↑ protein & caloric requirements with vitamin supplementation

        4) Excision of eschar to level of bleeding capillaries & split thickness skin grafts

        5) Marjolin's ulcer = squamous cell carcinoma arising in an ulcer or burn

F. ENT Trauma (Table 20)

TABLE 20	ENT Trauma*	
DIAGNOSIS	**Si/Sx's**	**TREATMENT**
Foreign body	1) Ear—insect in ear or object in ear. 2) Nose—persistent unilateral nasal drainage. 3) Airway—persistent pneumonia 4) Esophageal—3 most common areas of narrowing and lodging of foreign bodies a) Cervical Esophagus a) 16 cm from dental a) incisors b) Cardioesophageal level a) 23 cm from incisors c) Gastroesophageal jx a) 40 cm from incisors	1) ENT consult for extraction. Mineral oil in ear to kill insects while you wait. Don't irrigate vegetable matter or it will swell 2–4) ENT consult for extraction 1) CXR PA and lateral, and pulmonary or ENT consult for bronchoscopy and extraction. 2) CT scan of neck
Epistaxis	• Anterior bleed—most common 90% • Kiesselbachs plexus usually affected • Posterior bleed 10% • Nosebleeds can be life threatening	1) Airway, breathing, circulation 2) Calm patient and staff 3) Apply pressure, and consult ENT 4) Anterior bleed—silver nitrate cautery and/or nasal packing for 5 days with anti-staphylococcal prophylaxis 5) Posterior bleed—anterior and posterior pack or balloon 6) Surgical ligation or embolization of bleeding vessels is sometimes required
TM perforation	• Commonly occur after a slap in the face, or cotton swab in ear	• Po antibiotics and ear gtts • Water precautions

TABLE 20 *Continued*		
DIAGNOSIS	**Si/Sx's**	**Treatment**
Auricular hematoma	• Commonly seen in wrestlers. With repeated trauma to ears • Ecchymotic fluctuant fluid collection • If left untreated necrosis of auricular perichondrium can occur and patients develop a cauliflower ear	1) ENT consult 2) Incision and drainage of hematoma with drain left in place and Bolster dressing sutured in 3) Po antibiotics and careful follow-up
Nasal vestibulitis	1) Most commonly occurs after repeated rubbing of nose during URI or allergy season 2) Patients develop a cellulitis of nasal vestibule, which begins to spread along septum and dorsum of nose Because of valveless veins 3) draining this area of face, infection may spread to cavernous sinus and cause a cavernous sinus thrombosis patient to have visual changes, headache, or severe pain	1) Early on in infection may treat with po antibiotics and topical Mupirocin or bacitracin. Along with good nasal hygiene 2) If unsure, or non compliant patient, or sx's persist or worsen, admit for intravenous IV antibiotics 3) Maxillofacial/Orbital CT with contrast to rule out cavernous thrombosis may be needed
Blunt laryngeal trauma	• Hoarsness, stridor, voice changes, airway obstruction, subcutaneous emphysema, and hemoptysis	• ENT Consult. CXR, fiberoptic scope and CT Scan to evaluate injury and possible fracture • Airway observation in monitored setting. May need to secure airway (tracheostomy) • Humidified oxygen, and steroids. Surgery may be needed in severe trauma
Penetrating neck trauma	• Divided into three Zones • Zone 1—From sternal notch to cricoid cartilage Zone 2—Cricoid cartilage to angle of mandible • Zone 3—angle of mandible to skull base	• Zone 1 & 3—Surgical consult. Obtain Angiogram to evaluate extent of vascular involvement Zone 2—Surgical • exploration of wound or panendoscopy, angiography, esophagram, antibiotics and observation if patient is stable

TABLE 20	*Continued*	
DIAGNOSIS	**Si/Sx's**	**TREATMENT**
Nasal Fx	• There may be external and/or internal structural deviation • Must rule out septal hematoma/septal abscess to prevent ischemic compression of perichondrium and septal cartilage necrosis leading to saddle nose deformity • Evaluate for CSF leak • Repair any superficial lacerations	1) Any nosebleed should be stopped as described in Epistaxis 2) X-rays are not very helpful. Physical exam is all you need 3) ENT consult 4) Septal hematoma/abscess must be drained with a rubber drain left in place 5) Neurosurgery should be informed of potential CSF leak 6) Because of edema and severe pain most fracture (open or closed) reductions occur within 7–10 days in the O.R. under anesthesia if cosmesis or nasal airway is a concern 7) Antisthaphylococcus antibiotic prophylaxis given

Facial fracture	• LeFort fractures are the classic facial trauma fractures
	• Look for mobile palate (fractures always involve the pterygoid plates)
	1) Types of leFort fractures
	  a) LeFort 1 = maxilla fracture
	  b) LeFort 2 = pyramidal fracture on nasofrontal suture line
	  c) LeFort 3 = total craniofacial dysjunction
		• ENT/plastics/ or maxillofacial consult
		• Open vs. closed reduction with fixation devices (wiring vs. plating)

Mandible Fx	1) Most commonly affect the condyle, body and angle of mandible in that order 2) Multiple sites usually affected simultaneously 3) Sx's pain, malocclusion, trismus, crepitance, mucosal lacerations 4) Classsified as favorable if fracture fragments pull in the direction of splinting fracture. Unfavorable if forces on fracture line pull fragments apart	1) CT scan and panorex views are usually diagnostic 2) Antibiotics and pain meds needed 3) Open or closed reduction of fracture is needed and can be performed by oral surgery, plastics or ENT

TABLE 20	*Continued*	
DIAGNOSIS	**Si/Sx's**	**TREATMENT**
Temporal bone Fx	1) Transverse fractures—20% of fractures facial nerve involvement more likely and loss of hearing 2) Logitudinal—80% 3) Basilar skull fractures • Present with 4 classic physical findings: raccoon's eyes & Battle's sign, hemotympanum, CSF rhinorrhea and otorrhea a) Raccoon's eyes are dark circles (bruising) about the eyes, signifying orbital fractures b) Battle's sign is ecchymoses over the mastoid process, indicating a fracture there	• ENT and neurosurgery consult • Evaluate for CSF leak • Treat with antibiotic ear drops • IV antibiotics if CSF leak noted • May need immediate facial nerve decompression so status of facial nerve must be well documented • Audiogram needed to document status of cochlear nerve

*Note: All of the above conditions should be stabilized and evaluated by an Otorhinolaryngologist.

XXIV. HOARSENESS

A. Hoarseness (Dysphonia)

1. Perceived rough quality of the voice (caused by structural or functional abnormalities)

2. Many causes:

   a. **Congenital**—laryngeal webs, clefts, cysts

   b. **Infectious**—papillomatosis, viral, bacterial & fungal laryngitis, tuberculosis

   c. **Inflammatory**—reflux laryngitis, rheumatoid arthritis

   d. **Iatrogenic**—recurrent laryngeal nerve damage occurring during neck or cardiothoracic surgery

   e. **Traumatic**—vocal fold nodules, polyps, arytenoid dislocation, laryngeal framework disruption (fracture) and postintubation

   f. **Endocrine**—hypothyroidism, hyperthyroidism

   g. **Connective tissue disease**—scleroderma, sarcoidosis

h. **Neoplastic**

1) Benign—human papillomavirus, granuloma, laryngeal chondroma

2) Malignant (primary)—squamous cell carcinoma (larynx/lung) or thyroid cancer invading recurrent laryngeal nerve (RLN)

3) Malignant (metastasis)

i. **Neurologic**—vocal fold paralysis, multiple sclerosis, viral neuronitis, spasmodic dysphonia

j. **Senile larynx (old age)**
(Hoarseness differential by Dr. Ramon Franco, MEEI)

B. Larynx (Neoplasms)

1. Benign—most common is papilloma (human papillomavirus), chondroma, adenoma, chemodectoma (cherry red), and hemangioma

2. Malignant—squamous cell cancer most common

   a. Sx = hoarseness, stridor, otalgia, dyspnea, hemoptysis, weight loss, and adenopathy

   b. Tx = Surgery, chemotherapy, or radiation

XXV. COMMON ENT DRUGS (TABLE 21)

TABLE 21	Common ENT Drugs		
DRUG	**COMMON DRUGS**	**INDICATION**	**SIDE EFFECTS**
Antihistamines	• 1st Generation—benadryl, atarax • 2nd Generation—loratadine, fexofenedine, terfenadine, azelastin	Allergic rhinnitis, urticaria, atopic dermatitis, allergic disorders	• 1st Generation—Sedation, seizures, psychosis, anticholinergic effects • 2nd Generation—Mostly nonsedating, prolonged QT interval and torsades de pointes. Use with macrolide antibiotics, antifungals, SSRIs, and cimetidine is contraindicated

TABLE 21	Common ENT Drugs		
DRUG	**COMMON DRUGS**	**INDICATION**	**SIDE EFFECTS**
Decongestants	• Pseudophedrine, phenylephrine, oxymetazoline	Nasal congestion, sinusitis	• Severe rebound nasal congestion (rhinitis medicamentosa), hypertension, prostate enlargement, insomnia, appetite suppression
Ear preparations	• Antibiotics 1) Cortisporin® - Hydrocortison/ neomycin/poly-myxin 2) Ciprofloxacin Hydrocortisone 3) Ofloxacin	Otitis externa	• Neomycin known to cause erythematous skin reeaction in some patients
Nasal steroid sprays	• Budesonide-Rhinocort® • Fluticasone-Flonase® • Mometasone-Nasonex®	Allergic rhinitis	• Currently most effective treatment of allergic rhinnitis • Nosebleeds can occur if sprayed repeatedly onto septum

REVIEW QUESTIONS

1. Match the following symptoms with the appropriate diagnosis. Choices may be used only once

   1) A 25-yr-old female with a recent upper respiratory infection presents to the emergency room with severe continuous incapacitating vertigo lasting days. No hearing changes and no tinnitus

   a) Migraine

   2) A 40-yr-old female with severe headache, photophobia, and intermittent vertigo. No tinnitus, no hearing changes

   b) Benign positional vertigo

3) A 73-yr-old male with chronic progressive hearing loss, new onset intermittent tinnitus, and vertigo

c) Vestibular neuritis

4) A 56-yr-old male who c/o of severe vertigo lasting seconds when he gets out of bed in morning and whenever he goes to bed in evening

d) Acoustic neuroma

2. A young mother brings in her first baby for his 2-yr-old check up. During this visit she tells you that her child snores very loudly at night. He also has chronic nasal congestion and a very nasally voice. He constantly has his mouth open because he just can't breathe through his nose. He also is constantly having ear infections. No other symptoms. Choose the response that can most likely explain this patient's symptoms.

a) This patient obviously has significant sinus disease and must undergo endoscopic sinus surgery

b) This patient suffers from allergies and therefore must undergo immediate allergy workup and started on allergy shots

c) This patient has a benign condition and needs no intervention

d) The patient is most likely suffering from adenoiditis and should consider removal of adenoids

3. The patient in question 2 will be having surgery for their condition. What preoperative imaging study is indicated?

a) CT scan of the maxillofacial sinuses

b) MRI of head

c) Lateral neck film

d) Chest x-ray

4. Please match the following RED eye presentations with their associated diagnoses. Each choice may be chosen only once.

1) Sinus infection, periorbital erythema and edema

a) Angle closure glaucoma

2) Unilateral conjunctival erythema and pruritus

b) Subconjunctival hemorrhage

3) Bilateral conjunctival erythema and pruritus

c) Viral conjunctivitis

4) Recent weight lifting, erythema of conjunctiva, no pruritus

d) Allergic conjunctivitis

5) Pain, fixed mid-dilated pupil, blurry vision

e) Periorbital cellulitis

5. A 25-yr-old female presents to emergency room with a 1-wk hx of left-sided unilateral frontal headache unresponsive to oxycodone. Pt now developing left lid erythema, edema, and eye pressure. Pt denies any visual changes. Physical exam findings are consistent with above. CT scan consistent with frontal sinusitis and preseptal cellulitis. Choose the most appropriate treatment for this patient.

a) Continue oxycodone and discharge patient home on decongestants and nasal irrigations

b) Admit patient, give oral antibiotics, pain meds and decongestants

c) Admit patient, intravenous antibiotics, pain meds decongestants, nasal irrigation, possible surgery if symptoms continue to worsen

d) Discharge patient home, and follow up at general ENT clinic

6. A 76-yr-old male presents with new onset hoarseness and cough for the last week. Pt is a 1-pack-per-day smoker for the last 40 years, drinks a six pack of beer daily, and has a hx of gastroesophageal reflux. Fiberoptic examination of larynx reveals normal cord motion and open airway, and a question of mucosal changes on cords. Which of the following is most correct?

a) Patient most likely has senile larynx and therefore these finding are normal

b) Gastroesophageal reflux can commonly cause these symptoms so patient should be started on antacids and observed for improvement

c) Lung cancer and laryngeal cancer should be ruled out in this high risk patient. Obtain chest x-ray or CT scan of chest and neck, referral to ENT for panendoscopy and biopsy of mucosal changes

d) Patient is probably dehydrated from alcohol intake and with increased fluids will no longer be hoarse

7. A 24-yr-old female presents to emergency room with a 1-day hx of odynophagia, dysphagia, fever, and drooling.

No other sick contacts at home. Physical exam finds bilateral tonsillar hypertrophy, uvula midline, bilateral neck adenopathy, temp 100.2. Which of the following would your recommend for this patient?

a) Obtain throat culture, treat with amoxicillin for obvious strep infection. D/C home

b) Obtain ENT consult to rule out Lemierre's syndrome

c) Obtain lateral neck film, ESR, and CBC

d) Obtain Monospot, CBC, consider throat culture. Examine epiglottis with mirror. ENT consult if concerned for airway or peritonsillar abscess

8. Which bone makes up the medial wall of the orbit?

a) Ethmoid

b) Frontal

c) Palatine

d) Zygomatic

9. Which is **not** a feature of optic neuritis?

a) Slowly progressive vision loss

b) Disc hyperemia or edema

c) Pain on eye movement

d. Normal disc appearance

10. Which disorder presents as leucokoria?

a) Viral conjunctivitis

b) Scleritis

c) Angle closure glaucoma

d) Retinoblastoma

11. Which of the following is **not** a cause of congenital cataracts?

a) Rubella

b) Galactosemia

c) Amblyopia

d) Toxoplasmosis

12. Which is **not** a feature of age-related macular degeneration (AMD)?

a) Vision loss

b) Presence of choridal neovascular membranes

c) Hemorrhage

d) Pain

13. What is the most common orbital tumor in adults?

a) Capillary hemangioma

b) Cavernous hemangioma

c) Fibrous histiocytoma

d) Rhabdomyosarcoma

14. Which statement is false regarding corneal ulcers?

a) Does not occur in contact lens wearers

b) Causal organisms can be bacteria, virus, anaerobes, fungi

c) Can lead to vision loss

d) Can be associated with hypopyon

15. What is the first step in the care of patients with chemical burns?

a) Check vision

b) Steroids

c) Irrigation

d) Call ophthalmologist

ANSWERS

1. **1-c, 2-a, 3-d, 4-b.**

2. **d)** The patient may also have allergies but because of the repeated ear infections, and difficulty breathing at night, treating these allergies may not be enough. Therefore a lateral neck film should be done to evaluate the size of the child's adenoid pad and how much of the nasopharyngeal airway it actually occupies. If greater than 50% of the airway is occupied by adenoid or the patient has very significant symptoms then adenoidectomy is recommended. Sinus surgery would properly address this child's complaints.

3. **c)** As above.

4. **1-e, 2-c, 3-d, 4-b, 5-a.**

5. **c)** The possible spread of a frontal sinus infection to the brain and to the orbit warrant an admission with antibiotics, decongestants, nasal irrigation. Careful observation for changes in vision or mental status is absolutely indicated.

6. **c)** Lung cancer and laryngeal cancer should be ruled out in this high risk patient. Obtain chest x-ray or CT scan of chest and neck, referral to ENT for panendoscopy and biopsy of mucosal changes. Although it is possible that all the other choices may ultimately prove to be correct in a patient with so many risk factors, a careful and thorough workup for cancer is warranted and necessary.

7. **d)** Obtain Monospot, CBC, consider throat culture. Examine epiglottis with mirror. ENT consult if concerned for airway or peritonsillar abscess. Pt with mono are commonly treated with amoxicillin and later present scared with a rash all over their body. Therefore, it is reasonable to rule this out in patients. Whether or not to obtain a throat culture is controversial and most people treat for strep without obtaining cultures in order to prevent strep related disorders.
A patent airway is always a concern because many times pharyngeal swelling will extend downward and cause swelling of epiglottis and narrowing of patient's airway. These patients should be admitted for observation of airway and repeated endoscopic evaluation by ENT.

8. **a)** Medial wall composed of maxilla, lacrimal, ethmoid, and sphenoid bones, zygomatic bone part of lateral wall and floor of orbit. The frontal bone is part of the orbital roof and the palatine is a small bone in the posterior portion of the orbital floor.

9. **a)** Optic neuritis presents as an acute, abrupt, decrease in vision of variable severity. Slowly progressive vision loss is more typical of compressive optic neuropathy. Disc edema and hyperemia or a normal disc appearance can be seen in patients with optic neuritis. Often there is pain on eye movement.

10. **d)** Viral conjunctivitis, scleritis, and angle closure glaucoma commonly present with painful red eye. Viral conjunctivitis patients also have tearing, foreign body sensation, watery discharge, and preauricular adenopathy. Angle closure glaucoma patients have photophobia, blurry vision, and mid-dilated pupil. Patients with scleritis have severe pain with thinnning of sclera (blue in appearance due to underlying choroid). Leukocoria (white pupil) is commonly seen in children with retinoblastoma and also in cataracts.

11. **c)** Amblyopia can be caused by cataracts but is not a cause of congenital cataracts. Infections such as rubella, varicella, toxoplasmosis, and syphilis can cause congenital cataracts. Metabolic disorders such as galactosemia are also an etiology.

12. **d)** Pain is not a feature of AMD. Severe vision loss can occur, due to the presence of choroidal neovascular membranes leak and cause subretinal hemorrhages.

13. **b)** Cavernous hemangiomas are the most common orbital tumors in adults. Capillary hemangiomas are the most common orbital tumors in children. Fibrous histiocytoma is the most common mesenchymal tumors of adults. Rhabdomyosarcoma is the most common primary orbital malignancy in children.

14. **a)** Corneal ulcers often occur in contact lens wearers, secondary to poor lens hygiene and extended wear. Bacteria (*Pseudomonas, Moraxella*), viruses (herpes), fungi (fusarium) and parasites (acanthoamoeba) can cause ulceration with devastating vision loss. Hypopyon can occur in the setting of corneal ulcers, which is a poor prognostic sign.

15. **c)** Always irrigate first to remove the offending material. Visual prognosis is directly related to duration of chemical exposure to offending material. Remove any debris, and irrigate multiple times if needed. An ophthalmologist must then be called to evaluate patient and assist with visual exam.

INDEX

A

A-V nicking, 40t
ABCDE survey
  for ENT trauma, 130–132
  in malignant melanoma diagnosis, 116–117
Abscesses
  in otitis media, 63–64
  quinsy peritonsillar, 107
  retropharyngeal, 107
    treatment of, 108
Accommodation, ciliary muscle in, 6
Acetazolamide
  for glaucoma, 30
  uses and side effects of, 47t
Achalasia, 80–81
Achondroplasia, 57
Acoustic neuroma
  in asymmetric hearing loss, 70
  characteristics and treatment of, 72t
  diagnosis of, 141
Actinic keratosis, 117
Actinomyces israelii, 112
Acyclovir, 90
Adenocarcinoma, esophageal, 83
Adenoiditis, 112
  diagnosis and treatment of, 141, 144
Adenoids, enlargement of, 112f
Adenoma, thyroid, 125
Adenovirus
  characteristics, treatment, and diagnosis of, 113t
  throat, 106
Adie's tonic pupil, 16
Adrenergics, 46t
AEIOU TIPS, 131
African Burkitt's lymphoma, 120
Airway assessment, 130
Allergic conjunctivitis, 25t
Allergic hypersensitivity, 100
Alpha-agonists, 28
Alport's syndrome
  in hearing loss, 68
  ocular manifestations of, 41t
Amblyopia, 18, 146
Ameloblastoma, oral cavity, 102
Aminoglycoside, 88
Amoxicillin
  for otitis media, 63
  for sinusitis, 77t
Amphotericin, 77t
Anaplastic cancer, 129
Anesthetics, side effects of, 45t
Angioedema, 100–101

Angiofibroma, juvenile, 77
Anhidrosis, miotic pupils in, 17
Anisocoria, 16
Anopia
  inferior quadrantic, 10f
  superior quadrantic, 10f
Anosomia
  bilateral, 73
  unilateral, 73
Anterior chamber, embryology of, 4
Anti-Ro antibodies, 96
Anti-Smith antibodies, 96
Antibacterials, side effects of, 46t
Antibiotics
  for dacroadenitis, 33
  for dacryocystitis, 33
Anticholinergics, side effects of, 46t
Anticholinesterase inhibitors, 88
Antidepressants, 61t
Antihistamines, indications and side effects of, 139t
Antihistone antibodies, 97
Antinuclear antibody tests, 96
Antiphospholipid autoantibodies, 96–97
Antitumor necrosis factor antibody, 95
Antivirals, uses and side effects of, 46t
Apnea, during sleep, 110–111
Aqueous humor, 6
Argyll-Robertson pupil, 17
  medical conditions with, 41t
Arnold-Chiari malformation, 57
Arthritis, monoarticular, 67
Arthus reaction, 101
Artificial tears, 47t
Arytenoid cartilage, embryology of, 52t
Aspergillus infection
  in otitis externa, 62
  in sinusitis, 76
Aspirin, 128
Atarax, 139t
Atropine sulfate, 46t
Audiogram, 70
Auricular hematoma, 135t
Autoimmune diseases
  in hearing loss, 68
  in relapsing polychondritis, 66
  with uveitis, 27
Azathioprine
  for Crohn's disease, 95
  for myasthenia gravis, 88
  for Wegener's granulomatosis, 78
Azelastin, 139t
Azithromycin, 63

P